Yesterday's Dentistry

*Voices from the British Dental Association
Oral History Archive*

Andrew Sadler

With the voices of:

Barbara Huntley, William Patterson, Alan Mayhew, Laurence Oldham, Oliver Gowers, Professor Sir Paul Bramley, Alan Seaton, Gordon Fordyce, Peter Kaspar, Freda Rimini, Stuart Robson, John Bayes, Bernadette Rivett, Douglas Johnston, Russell Hopkins, Shelagh Farrell, Roy Walton, Barry Devonald, Barry Cockcroft, Ron Broadway, Dolly Terfus, Philip Sutcliffe, John Beal, Michael Butterworth, Eva Milburn, Roland Hopwood, Robin Addis, Stanley Gelbier, Nigel Williams, Leslie Cheeseman.

Yesterday's Dentistry

Voices from the British Dental Association Oral History Archive

ISBN: 978-1-7393838-0-0

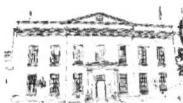

BROKESLEY HOUSE   2023

Contents

******

Preface

The story told here starts in the 1940s before the start of the National Health Service.

Before and after WWII, dental health in Britain was appalling. Dental caries and periodontal disease were rife. Oral hygiene measures were practised only by the prosperous and some of the middle classes. Toothbrushes were expensive items not bought by the so-called working classes. For many the first time they had a toothbrush was when they were recruited into the armed forces.

Dentists were nearly always male. Most had qualified with the LDS diploma from one of the Royal Colleges of Surgeons but there were still registered dentists who had received no formal training. Anyone practising and earning their main income from dentistry for five of the seven years preceding the 1921 dentist act could register, so could dental mechanics. There were only a few dentists qualified with a university degree.

Restorative dentistry was difficult without high-speed drills and modern burs and, when used, amalgam was mixed by hand. For many, multiple extractions and full dentures made of vulcanite, a form of rubber, was the only dentistry they received; or perhaps, was the only treatment the dentist could do.

Most dentists operated from their own homes. They usually had a single surgery and waiting room and lived above the practice. They may have employed a dental mechanic in the basement.

This book contains stories of how this changed and is told by dental professionals who practised from this time. They were interviewed, and the recordings transcribed between 2011 and 2023, as part of the British Dental Association, John McLean history archive, often, but not exclusively, in the subjects' homes. The recordings were made on broadcast quality equipment in a lossless format and were transcribed literally, i.e. exactly as spoken. The copyright of the original recordings is held by the British Dental Association.

The transcriptions have been heavily edited to remove repetition, deviation, and unnecessary words into a readable text.

Andrew Sadler   September 2023

1. Barbara Huntley

Barbara remembers having orthodontic treatment in the 1930s and becoming a dental assistant in Ruislip in 1946. She describes the work of two practices she worked in and the change when the National Health Service started in 1948. Barbara was interviewed by Stephen Simmons at the British Dental Association headquarters in 2011.

******

Orthodontic treatment 1930s.

My mother took me to King's College, and I can remember the part of the building now. It wasn't where the present one is. The chairs actually faced Ruskin Park. I can remember the long corridors, and there were lots of central heating pipes running through them. I had a frenectomy done there, which is done if you have a diastema, a big space between your teeth. My mother had a very large space between her central teeth and didn't want me to have the same.

Then I followed it with orthodontic treatment, and I remember my four lower front incisors were covered with a silver cap. I'm not too sure for what reason, but they were. And I remember going to school and the children had seen nothing like it, so they were all looking in my mouth to see this cap. And after that the war broke out and life changed for everybody, so I had no more treatment. It was 1939.

Orthodontic treatment was very rare then and it was only because my mother bothered to take me. I don't think I was referred by anybody because I don't think you had to get referred in those days. We didn't even go to the doctor. I think you had to pay to go to the doctor, and we were very poor. My father died when I was five and we had so little money.

Dental nursing 1945

I was born in Brockley, South London, but I grew up in Catford until the war. When the house was bombed, we moved to Ruislip, in Middlesex, and I went to Harrow County Girls' School.

It was 1945 when I left school and I wanted to be a nurse, but my mother wasn't keen. She probably thought it was too tough a life. At 16, I was too young anyway. Just by chance, I saw an advert in the paper for a dental assistant in Ruislip so I applied and got the job. As it turned out, I enjoyed it and carried on for most of my working life doing that. When my children had more or less grown up, I did do general nursing training, so I got my wish after all.

Strangely the dentist I worked for in Ruislip was German, as were his wife and mother-in-law. I've only now wondered how the German dentist was working there.

He was extremely nice, and his family. Not long afterwards, we had to move back to Catford, and they didn't want me to go, so they asked if I would like to stay with them during the week, and go back home weekends. I did that for a time but it wasn't particularly good for a young person, so after about a year I went go back to my original home in Catford.

I quickly got a job with a practice in New Cross, which was a tram ride away in those days. The practice in Ruislip had been very modern with up-to-date equipment but the New Cross practice was very old-fashioned, but I adapted to it and the dentist was very nice. That was when the National Health came in.

The work was mostly extractions and dentures. The war had not long finished, rationing was still in, and people had never been to a dentist for years. It was a very poor neighbourhood, and it was a time of upheaval, so people's mouths were in pretty poor condition, so it was mostly extractions. We did a lot of extractions under anaesthetic, which the doctor used to come for.

The dentist was excellent at replacement dentures. They still had a choice of vulcanite, or if they could afford it, they would have acrylic. We had lots of vulcanite dentures with the rubber suction disc on the top, which cost seven shillings and sixpence.

We didn't have a steriliser, we just had blue glass jars with Lysol in them, which I changed every day. I washed the forceps and put them in.

The Ruislip practice must have been quite new because it was extremely up to date, and we certainly had a steriliser there, and a very modern gas machine The one in New Cross was just, more or less, two cylinders and two rubber bags on wheels which we pushed into the surgery.

Everything was very basic. We had a long and a short needle which were only changed once a day, and every patient shared them. They were placed into the Lysol in the jar, which is unthinkable now. I just accepted it, and nothing ever went wrong, which is quite surprising. I don't recall we ever stopped using only two needles a day. We certainly never wore gloves, or any other sort of prevention.

One day, I stabbed my thumb with a dirty needle, and I got a nasty sore thumb, but I put some spirit on it, and it helped. I never got Hepatitis C or anything. I remained healthy throughout.

The dentist was excellent at extractions, because most of the work was extractions and always had been. He was quite elderly when I got there, so his experience, past and present, was of extractions and replacements. We did fillings, but we didn't do crowns. We did gold fillings, the best ones were gold foil, and I still think they're good.

I would mix the alloy and the mercury up in a little glass pestle and mortar, then put it into my hand and knead it, wring it out in the cloth. You wouldn't think now of touching mercury, would you? And I did that for years, and I never got mercury poisoning.

General anaesthetic extractions were always at lunchtime, the last patient before lunch. I would ring up the doctor, who lived not very far away, and he would come along and give the anaesthetic. I would stand there with the enamel kidney dish; I can remember the ping ping as each tooth went into it. We never ever had a calamity; nothing ever went wrong. The doctor was very affable; he was pleased to come, and he got paid cash in hand. After, the patient stayed in the chair because they were the last patient of the morning. I'd look after them they would sit with a pack in their mouth till they stopped bleeding, and then we'd give them instructions.

The practice was in a family house, so the big front room was the waiting room as you came in the front door, and the back room was the surgery, and the rest of the house was private. The telephone was just outside in the hall. It worked well, although it was old-fashioned.

If the phone went, I'd take the appointment book outside, and the dentist seemed to manage without me. I'm sure, until I arrived, his wife had done the work, but she really wasn't well and I think I was the first assistant he'd ever had. It was quite unusual in those days to have a paid assistant, because it was usually the wife that just opened the door and let them in, and probably the dentist mixed his own fillings. That was the way it was until the National Health came in and then, of course, everything changed.

We had an X-ray machine, and I used to develop them in the bathroom at the back. I think the quality of the X-rays was as good as they would be even today. Although everything was antiquated, it seemed to work very well. The patients were always happy, and loads of them just came back repeatedly and brought their children with them. But, of course, nobody knew any different anyway, and I think people were so relieved the war was over, that people were really nice and grateful for what they had.

The biggest and most frequent complications were dry sockets, which caused the patient a lot of pain. But it was easily rectified. We syringed it with some disinfectant, probably peroxide. The patient would come back a few times, and be given instructions on mouth wash, and they would clear up. I'm sure they were caused because some of the patients' mouths had been terrible for so long and it was, sometimes, inevitable they were going to get trouble afterwards. They had had no education about looking after teeth and keeping them clean in the normal way. People were really very poor in 1930s, which were pretty grim, and then straight away, the war, so it was really a very long period of deprivation.

The practice was private when I went there; the patients paid for their treatment. I think it was seven shillings and sixpence to take a tooth out. And we did an awful lot of denture repairs. There was a dental technician, an elderly man and a young boy assistant, who worked downstairs in the basement, so we could do repairs quickly. They obviously made the dentures as well, so they would pop up during the day to show the dentist how it was going and I popped down, to see how long would they would take to do a repair. It worked very well. It was an awful lot about dentures in those days.

National Health Service practice in south London late 1940s

When the National Health started in 1948, we were much busier, and the vast majority of the work was clearances, removing all the patient's teeth. If we could, we left something, especially in at the bottom, to retain the lower denture, which is normal practice, and even in the upper if we could. Before people didn't have regular dental treatment. Mostly they couldn't afford it or it wasn't available even. People's mouths were in a terrible state so they were so pleased to have their bad teeth extracted. And if they could afford it, they had an immediate temporary denture, which I'm pretty sure they had to pay for themselves. I don't think the

National Health paid for temporary dentures, I can't really remember. The majority had temporary dentures for some months until their mouths had settled down, and then they would have their permanent ones fixed.

A relief for the dentist was that we didn't have to ask the patients for money. I just had to sit there filling up EC17s like mad. I think everybody was happy with the situation. We could certainly cope. We didn't do crowns and all the fancy treatments that would take a lot of time. It was relatively easy to do fillings, and we did scalings.

I think the dental chair originally had been one of the very early moquette types, and had been re-upholstered into leather. It was, even to me then, very old-fashioned. But, as basic as it was, it really worked. We had an operating light to move about. The drill was powered with electricity, it wasn't pedalled. I think there was a pedalled drill downstairs in the laboratory which was used for the dentures. The dentures often needed a lot of adjusting.

We used to get our equipment and everything from Cottrell's in Charlotte Street. When we needed anything, I'd give them a ring, and they'd deliver it, and the same for the oxygen company. When we needed cylinder replacements, I'd give them a ring, and it would come.

We gave advice about hygiene, particularly after extractions, salt mouthwash, always salt. Certainly not diet advice, because remember rationing was still on, so there wasn't much point. He didn't do any orthodontics or root canal treatment. I never remember anybody being referred for treatment. Perhaps they had been, but I don't recall that at all.

We started at ten; we had a break for lunch, and I remember we always had a drink mid-morning. The dentist's wife was very kind. She always brought me up a cup of tea or something, and frequently it was Bovril. And I loved that, the Bovril. And then we started work again, and we worked, I think until six, and then had another, I think the dentist had his tea then, but we carried on working till eight o'clock, but we had Wednesdays off, which was very nice. I didn't mind getting home late too much. We worked till about six on Saturday, and then eventually we cut down a bit, maybe till four on a Saturday. The dentist was getting older, he wasn't a young person, and his wife died, so that changed things. I remember I used to make the tea for him.

I worked there from about early 1946 to 1953. And that was when I left to have my children.

National Health Service practice late 50s and 60s

By 1957, I'd had two children, and I was living in Brixton, and I found a practice that worked in the evenings, so I worked from six till nine o'clock every evening, and later Saturdays as well.

That was a very interesting practice, because there were so many dentists. We had a day shift, and then a night shift, at six o'clock. Most of the dentists that came were newly qualified from King's College Hospital, which was very close.

The dental nurses dealt with the paperwork, the appointments and absolutely everything, so the dentist had nothing to do except look after his patient. And for a newly qualified person with really no experience of being a dentist in the outside world, it worked extremely well. We were mostly about the same age, but we also got some older dentists. I worked with an Australian dentist for a long time, they were all nice and we all got on all right. There was a practice manager and I think, nine surgeries, so it was extremely busy. We had a very large laboratory in the back, down the garden.

I was there for quite a long time. I left in 1972 to do general nursing. And sometimes during that time I would be asked if I could just fill in while a regular nurse was going on holiday. Also, I went to Chelsea and did a stint every year, and I can remember going to Ealing to somebody else.

I really enjoyed my days as a dental nurse and certainly met some very interesting people. And then in the middle, I managed to do my general nursing too, which was made very much easier by the previous experience I'd had. It gave me the confidence, and I could respond to the patients in the hospital because I was used to them. I have no regrets about what I've done. I've done a bit of both, that's very nice. I retired from dental nursing in 1998 when I was nearly 70, that was because the dentist I was working for retired as well.

2. William Patterson

William qualified in Belfast in 1946 and was a General Dental Practitioner in Northern Ireland at the start of the National Health Service. He spoke to Judith Painter in 2016.

*****

I trained at Queen's University Belfast Dental School from 1941 to 1946. We started off with 12 students and after one year six of them had dropped out, leaving six of us. To study dentistry, you required a senior certificate or equivalent.

Mostly extractions in Londonderry

When I finished dentistry, I went to Londonderry and did a locum for a year. There were about six or seven dentists practising and they were all quite elderly, but when the health scheme started in 1948, new dentists came in and there were no problems in getting patients.

The Derry people were very poor. Most of their money came from the ladies who worked in the shirt factories. The men were unemployed and spent their time drinking and gambling, dentistry was a very low priority. But after the health scheme came, the treatment was free and most of them then had teeth extracted, but until then very few of them went to a dentist.

Before the NHS patients had to pay for treatment, but the charges weren't very high, but there was no money available in Londonderry for dental treatments. Most of the work was extractions, clearances. Some were done with local anaesthetic, there were no anaesthetists available, but the doctor came in and gave an anaesthetic when a lot of extractions were required. After the extractions, I would provide them with dentures, but I did not have a dental technician, so I sent them out to one that was available in Londonderry. There were very few technicians available and any difficult cases were sent to the Dental School in Belfast, a two-hour journey.

Second-hand electric drill

The health scheme started in 1948 and I started up on my own in a rented house. Most of the dentists worked from their own home where they had surgery and waiting rooms. They had a receptionist and perhaps a part-time assistant. I worked standing up with a second-hand electric drill, but when they became available, I purchased a new unit, that was about 1951. My family had money so I did not require a loan from the bank.

Acrylic replacing vulcanite and arrival of air rotor drill

We started off training with the vulcanite dentures and then, when acrylic dentures came on the market, we changed to acrylic. The fillings were usually amalgam for the posterior teeth and white synthetic for the front teeth but as time went on the materials improved and, of course when the high-speed drill was invented it revolutionised all forms of dental treatment, crowns, bridges, etc. That was about 1950/60s. Before that we used the electric drill; we would spend 30 minutes on one filling. So, the high-speed drill was really terrific, plus the new materials.

I didn't do many crowns at the beginning but with the new equipment and the new high-speed drill crowns became more common and the patients were quite willing to have them done. At that stage, they had to pay a bit on the National Health.

Then I got a chair so I could sit down to work but I preferred to stand up. I stood up for most of the time and I wore a white coat. There was a steriliser, and that was with boiling water. I usually tried to use a new needle for each patient, but if the needle was used twice, it was sterilised.

When the anaesthetists became available in the 1950s, I employed one. The local hospital had no dental surgery, but when the Altnagelvin Hospital was built in late 1950s or 1960 there was a dental department there and available for patients that gave trouble, difficult cases.

I did some root canal work for front teeth. They weren't always successful, but you did your best. I had to send the patients to the local hospital for X-rays, as I did not have an X-ray machine for several years, but once an X-ray machine was on the market, I purchased one and that made it so much easier.

I knew some other dentists but there's only one or two that I was really friendly with. The British Dental Association had monthly meetings, but they weren't very helpful. The NHS made a big difference;

we had forms to fill in and patients signed and they sent down another dentist to check over your work to see that it was up to standard.

When the Troubles came, that made a difference. Patients from the other side of the city side could not keep appointments on account of the bombing. That was in the 1970s.

Education played a part in the improvement. People weren't aware of the value of their teeth and, through time they became aware and made regular appointments. That education was from the dentists, and I suppose publicity in the papers.

3. Alan Mayhew

Alan Mayhew started dentistry during WWII in 1942 at Guy's. He told how the preclinical students were evacuated to Tunbridge Wells and he had to work part time in the fire service. Later a BDS exam was interrupted by a bomb landing nearby. His interest in surgery followed a visit to East Grinstead and later his work at Rooksdown House. He was interviewed by Stephen Simmons in 2011

******

During the war, I was living with my parents down in Worthing outside of the blitz area of London. Little did we know Hitler would arrive on the other side of the channel a year later. The dentist I went to as a young student was a Guy's man and I had, I think, 18 visits on one occasion and 16 on another, and locals took a long time to work and my teeth were absolutely rotten. So, he had a lot of time to chat with me and as a result of that I got interested in dentistry.

I began my training at Guy's in 1942. I went to Sherwood Park in Tunbridge Wells to do my first MB examination.[1] We were a small group. BDS was just coming in to popularity as a university degree. Most people were doing LDS, the old RCS exam.[2]

When I started doing dentistry, all teeth were porcelain with little pins in the back of them which were then processed into vulcanite dentures. When I started doing my prosthetic training, which is five terms in Guy's, I was learning to make vulcanite dentures. But by the time I finished poly methyl methacrylate, the acrylic resin had come in and we were making dentures in plastic. And this, of course, was an area John McLean was

---

[1] Sherwood Park, near Tunbridge Wells contained an Italianate mansion constructed in the 1860s. At the start of WWII it was taken over by Guy's Hospital for use by the Dental School. It was demolished in 1995 to make way for housing.

[2] The first Bachelor of Dental Surgery degrees in England were awarded in Birmingham in 1906. The first qualification in dentistry was the Licentiate in Dental Surgery of the Royal College of Surgeons of England in 1860 See: Gelbier S. 125 years of developments in dentistry, 1880–2005. Part 5: Dental education, training and qualifications. British Dental Journal, 199 (2005) 10 685 - 689.

very interested in, apart from the advances on silicates which were the rather poor-quality anterior fillings we had to use in those days.

Preclinical studies and being evacuated during the war

Because the war was on, the pre-clinical people were evacuated from London. I was in Sherwood Park. There was a warden, Professor Fenn, who was the Professor of Prosthetics. There were two others, one was Hurstmead, another big house where Professor Spurrell, the Physiologist, was warden. I think they called them wardens.

So, we had this complex of three places and our lectures were given down at the Baptist Tabernacle in Tunbridge Wells. Because we were 'reserves' doing medicine and dentistry, we all had to be involved in either the home guard or you could apply to go into the fire service.[3] My memory of being in the in OTC, Officer Training Corps, at school was crawling through heather and such like and getting my knees rather sore on field days. And waving flags and shooting blanks, so I went into the fire service.

Students working in the fire service

We had a trailer, an old Trojan lorry and a 250cc Coventry Climax pump. The only fire we ever attended was when we set our own trailer on fire. You had to tickle the carburettor and swing the handle and a magneto would cause sparks and we over-tickled the carburettor, so we had a fire on our trailer. There was no fire extinguisher on the trailer and the nearest hydrant for our hoses was miles away. We were a little team, there were six of us, we used to spend the night at weekends down at the local fire service; we weren't popular with the regulars.

We were all living together, three to a room, in this house at Sherwood Park. Professor Fenn called us together one night and said 'There's been a proposal at Guy's, which I have to put to you, that we might take ladies on the dental course.' Well, I have to tell you there was a full 'no' vote. But the following year, six young ladies joined the dental course.

Bombed during BDS exam

One day I was doing one of my BDS exams in South Kensington, at a place called Jehangir Hall. It was just behind the Science Museum. We were at folding desks with ink wells because the biros hadn't got to us in those days.

---

[3] Students in medicine and dentistry was considered to be in 'reserved' occupations that could not be called up for military service and were not allowed to volunteer.

We were being invigilated by a series of clergymen, who were up on the stage where they were standing around when a V1 stopped popping, and we all looked at one another and all we could do was to crouch under our folding desks, and this thing landed in the corner of the Natural History Museum on the Cromwell Road and went off.

We were shielded from the direct blast by the Science Museum but the actual earth shake caused the dust of ages to come out of the hammer beam roof of the hall and our ink wells popped up and down on the folding desks. The invigilators looked like a series of crows diving, their gowns going up behind them as they dived under the grand piano. I can remember so clearly. We were given a ten percent discount on the pass mark on that exam. And I thank Hitler for that V1.

We were working late one evening in the laboratory at Guy's, there were three of us, and there was an almighty bang and roar and we dived on the floor. The glass came all over us and it was a V2 on this occasion. It landed in Nettleford's in the Borough High Street. And we got up, brushed ourselves down, no injury, and went home. You just got on with it.

Surgeon breaks jaw at East Grinstead

One thing we were given as students was a trip to East Grinstead. Sir William Kelsey Fry, one of the senior dental surgeons at Guy's, used to go down there. There were four main oral surgeons at East Grinstead during the war, and the students were given a day's trip down to watch the goings on. I can well remember the day that we visited, sitting in the gallery of the operating theatre at East Grinstead and Sir William Kelsey Fry was working away with his hammer and mallet and fractured the jaw of a patient he was operating on. He turned round to look at us and he said, 'And there, gentlemen, you can see how easy it is to break a jaw.' He took off his gown and left the registrar to wire the patient up and he came and gave us a lecture. Well, I must admit, it was probably that day that I decided I would not go on with restorative dentistry and my career lay in hospital. I wanted to go into hospital work.

I won three of the prizes in the prosthetics years and I was up for the Newland Pedley prize.[4] I'd put my name forward for it and John McLean was doing it as well; we competed with one another. Now, I was already

---

[4] Named after Frederick Newland-Pedley (1855-1944) who became dental surgeon at Guy's Hospital in 1887 and founded the dental department and dental school which opened in 1889.

losing enthusiasm for a future in restorative dentistry and the better man won. John got the Newland Pedley prize.

Rooksdown House

I came back to Guy's after my service in the air force and Martin Rushton had been my first chief after he came out of the war service. He suggested I went down to Rooksdown House and do six months there. So, I went to Rooksdown House which is down in Basingstoke. It was one of the units set up by Sir Harold Gillies, who'd worked with Sir William Kelsey Fry in the First World War.[5]

I was promised six months there, but I got so interested that I stayed for three years. I used to assist this man who I found a fascinating character, and that's why I ended up no longer having an enthusiasm for doing West End dentistry. When I came back from Rooksdown I worked for three years with Alan Thomson in Harley Street, part-time and learnt that I didn't want to do that.

Well, I suppose in my life, the great thing was that Martin Rushton sent me to Rooksdown House. Because having worked there for three years, I never lost touch with the patients and, Sir Harold Gillies. He followed an example set by Archie McIndoe, who had formed a club for these burned airmen at East Grinstead. There the nurses used to take them in to East Grinstead to mingle with the public because it was more than the burns which affected these people. It was the mental disability as well, which the trauma of the injuries left on them.[6]

Gillies saw the advantages of this and we formed a similar club but broader spectrum called the Rooksdown Club. I say broader spectrum because it involved civilians who were involved in wartime injuries and

---

[5] Rooksdown House was a large house in the grounds of Park Prewett mental hospital, Basingstoke, which was used for the private patients. It was taken over by the Emergency Medical Service during WWII for the treatment of facial injuries. In 1948 when the National Health Service started it became the Regional Centre for Plastic Surgery and Jaw Surgery for the South West Metropolitan Region, which it remained until 1959 when the unit was moved to Queen Mary Hospital, Roehampton. For an in- depth description of Rooksdown House in WWII see: Millar, Simon 2015 Rooksdown House and the Rooksdown Club: A Study into the Rehabilitation of Facially Disfigured Servicemen and Civilians Following the Second World War. Doctoral thesis, University of London. Available to download at: https://sas-space.sas.ac.uk/6264/ (Sourced March 2023).
[6] Martin Amsler Rushton (1903-1970) had worked as a dental surgeon at Rooksdown House during the war and became Dean of Guy's dental school. His main clinical interest became oral medicine and pathology. See: Plarr's Lives of the Fellows. Royal College of Surgeons (on line).

after the war, car injuries. And that Rooksdown Club has gone on until last year,[7] it's followed me around, I've followed patients all this time, because coming to Wessex I came back into the centre where a lot of the patients live.

---

[7] He was speaking in 2011.

4. Laurence Oldham

Laurence described in detail being a dental student in Birmingham in the early 1950s including an alcoholic pub crawl, by car, to Stratford-upon-Avon. He worked as a dentist in practice and in the RAF in National Service in the RAF and after a 'boring' academic job became an oral and maxillofacial surgeon. Laurence spoke to me at his home in Taunton in 2012.

******

My parents took my sister to Birmingham Dental Hospital for orthodontic treatment. I can remember going with the family up the stairs to the orthodontic department, and I had one of those rare flashes of insight. This is what I want to do. And from that day on I showed an interest in hospital work.

Failure to get into medical school

I applied to medical school first, but I came out of the secondary education in 1949-50. There were a lot of ex-forces people in the market for university places, and they were much more mature and I think the interview panel in medicine realised that here was a relatively insignificant newcomer straight from school and wasn't really up to the medical course. Because of that rejection, I decided on dentistry.

Undergraduate dentistry

We had a manual dexterity test. We had to bend wire into the professor's initials, J O, John Osborne, who seemed to be in charge of the interviews. And then we had to carve an incisor from a cube of wax. When I finished, with about 25 others, I looked around and some of them were very good indeed, beautifully artistic wire bending for J O and very authentic carving for teeth. Mine were rather mediocre, I'm afraid to say at that stage, because I hadn't really developed much manual skill.

I got an offer which seemed to be unconditional, providing I'd got through A-levels. I'd read physics, chemistry and biology. Biology I did as a cram subject because we didn't have biology in the boys' school. So, it was very exciting to go across the road to the girls' school and do biology with the girls.

I started in 1950 in Birmingham. I applied to the lodgings officer who fixed me up in Selly Park Road, which was a very nice tree lined dormitory area about a mile away from Edgbaston and the medical school. It was an ideal situation. Mr and Mrs Pilling were the proprietors, she ran the house. There was a Norwegian on the upper floor studying chemistry. There were six of us on the second floor, some medical students, some further chemistry students, and then there were some much older men who weren't at the university at all. They'd remained after finishing their university degrees as lodgers, so it was a very mixed house and very interesting.

I learned an awful lot from everybody in this house for the first year. And then Mrs Pilling developed some terrible cardiac problem, and the place had to close. So I was given the job of finding a place where all these people could live. I went round to another part of Edgbaston and found a place that would take us all. It wasn't very successful because it was run by two Scottish people who were very keen on tidiness. There were regulations posted on the back of the bedroom doors, and this went down badly with our group. We'd been used to freedom in Mrs Pilling's place. It was a very happy setup at Mrs Pilling's. This was too big a contrast, and we all split up into various places after that.

Most of my classmates were much older than me because they had been in the forces. I think half were ex-forces. We had one captain from the Indian army, Captain Donovan. But we had people from the army, navy and air force, and they seemed to us very mature and they knew how to study. Some of us from school, myself particularly, didn't really know how to study at all and there was a big difference between A-level work when you could be coached in the subject and you go to the exam knowing more or less what the questions might be, whereas university teaching was totally different. I hadn't really grasped this difference in the early stages.

In the first year, we were in the same lecture hall as the medical students. We were a combined medical and dental course and we had lectures on physiology from Professor Golding and lectures on anatomy. Then we separated into discreet lectures for dental students, which were taken by a surgical registrar called Bevan, who was very good. He was very clever at drawing on the blackboard, say the carotid artery tree, he could draw this beautifully and name all the branches of the external carotid and all the nerve pathways. We didn't have overhead projectors, slides or anything like that then. It was all done with a blackboard and chalk, and cleverly too. The first year was basic science with the medical students and we joined in the lab work with them, with the frog's legs muscles, action potentials for nerves. We did all the basic physiology for the medical course, the same.

In the second year, we then went to the dental laboratory course, which was again in the medical school on the second floor. We each had our own station with a peg that you could work on in the middle of the desk arrangement, and a drawer underneath and a flat surface to do your prosthetic mock-ups on. It was all to do with prosthetics, how to mix plaster, how to wax up and flask a denture, how to get the right teeth, mould, shape, size, bite blocks, how to make bite blocks, how to register a bite. Total prosthetic laboratory procedures really, flasking, burning out the wax, casting the acrylic, compressing the acrylic, waiting for it to set.

Then we left the medical school and went down into the centre of town to Great Charles Street. In Great Charles Street, we started off in a prefab building which was the Op. Tech. course and we had phantom heads and treadle drills. Each student had a station with a treadle drill rather like a Singer sewing machine worked by foot, with a series of arms and cords, and on the end, you could put an old-fashioned hand piece. And then we had phantom heads which you had teeth set into plaster and we had to do cavities on these teeth. I remember it was quite hazardous because of the dentine dust. We were not given any protective masks or anything to wear, and we must have all inhaled this dentine and enamel dust over quite a protracted period.

I remember we had a very critical teacher called R.J. Smith who wouldn't let anything through at all. Every student had to go through to his office with your phantom head and show what you'd done with the latest, say it was an MOD cavity preparation. You had to take it through and show R.J. Smith, who had a loop. He would examine every aspect of this MOD preparation. He would point out that the angles were wrong, if they were, or the depth was wrong or it was too near the pulp. It was tremendous heavy criticism which stayed with me for the rest of my career. Somehow, I built into myself a super critical faculty of the work I was doing. You couldn't help it. Before you saw R.J. Smith, after the first month or so you examined your own stuff in the most minute detail to get it passed by him. And blow me, he would still always find some fault. He was a real stickler for exactitude.

In our third year, when we got through the Op. Tech. course and R.J. Smith's inquisitorial approach, when he felt we were able to, we went up to room six in the Birmingham Dental Hospital. Room six had about 25 to 30 chairs in several rows. We were given a list of patients which we called in. So that's when we started our conservative work on patients.

In year four, we were surgical dressers and rotated down to the general hospital in Steelhouse Lane, Birmingham General Hospital. That's where I had a second flash of insight because as dressers, we were required to give anaesthesia for general surgical problems like breast abscesses or paraphymoses. We gave anaesthetics, under supervision, while the medical students did the surgery. And this, I found, was the most exciting thing I'd ever done. It was a throwback to my original inkling to do medicine. This was the nearest I came to doing medicine. And I look back on those dresser days, rotating out to the general hospital with great satisfaction and interest and enjoyment. That was really what I wanted to do.

R.J. Smith in Op. Tech influenced the whole of the rest of my career. But now in the dental hospital itself, there was D.B. Wells who was another finick who wanted everything absolutely perfect. So, everybody tried to avoid him and went to Mrs Hoggins, who was an easier touch to get anything passed. Again, we had to get everything checked: cavities, lining, filling, polishing, presentation. And I can see my fellows were trying to choose which demonstrator would let them through, but of course there wasn't always the same choice of demonstrator. Sometimes you had to have D.B. Wells, who was very awkward. But it all made for better standards really.

In Oral Surgery we were taught by Mr Brown, Father Brown he was known as. He took us one at a time in a single room with a patient and he would always loosen the tooth with a straight elevator before we were allowed to extract the tooth. We never approached a virgin tooth to extract it unless he'd loosened it with an elevator. Always under local anaesthesia. He would guide us in the extraction technique. It was one-to-one with a succession of patients and we had a lot of teeth to extract. There was a lot of caries after the war. I can't ever remember doing surgical extractions, just did straightforward extractions. Father Brown – he was very elderly – was such a good extractor so I don't honestly ever remember breaking a tooth. If we did, he would get the bits out without doing a flap, he would somehow manage to get them out. We didn't do impacted wisdom teeth at all.

Pub crawl and incident in Stratford

I'm not proud of this incident, but with all these ex-forces in the year, I was led astray on a pub crawl to Stratford-on-Avon. In those days, in the 1950s, many of us drove. I wasn't a driver, but I joined a group, four of us, in a Ford Popular. We drove in a whole convoy of cars from Birmingham to Stratford on a pub crawl, stopping at various pubs; however we did it I don't know.

By the time we got to Stratford, we were all practically oiled. I remember entering The Swan and tripping on a ledge on the floor halfway down the corridor, just after purchasing a pint of beer. It was late in the evening and Dennis Sadler was sitting on the floor in the corridor, with his legs out in front of him, just smiling benignly. As I tripped, I emptied the whole pint on the top of his bald pate and I can't remember him showing any displeasure or irritation at all. I was very apologetic because it hadn't been intentional, but Dennis seemed to take it as a matter of routine.[8]

The LDSRCS. exam

I went to London as an external candidate to the LDSRCS because I thought that would be valuable in coming up to qualification from Birmingham.[9] I was very well versed in the basic science, medicine and anatomy. I got through the LDSRCS part one straightaway, which was quite thrilling because I came back to Birmingham having got through that and then sat the BDS later.

The LDSRCS part one was the written work and then the second part was we were examined with a viva in London. I don't remember any clinical work, but certainly we were examined with quite a searching viva. I was asked to delineate the tumours from the elementary tract starting from the mouth, through to the anus, which I was able to do. And the examiner seemed quite happy with that, so I got through that and went back to Birmingham to do the BDS. And I specialised for six months in oral surgery. Every BDS student had to do some specialty, either restorative or oral surgery or periodontology. I chose oral surgery because of the experience in the general hospital inclined me towards surgery right from the start.

---

[8] In 2012 when I interviewed Laurence, I confessed that Dennis Sadler was my uncle. Laurence never saw him after this incident and I explained that he was chucked out after failing the 2nd BDS exam. I was able to tell him that Dennis later passed the College of Surgeons 2nd LDS exam and then did clinical training in Sheffield, where he was a model student, or so he said.

[9] Licentiate in Dental Surgery of the Royal College of Surgeons. The first qualification in dentistry in the UK started in 1860. See: S. Gelbier. 125 years of developments in dentistry, 1880–2005 Part 5: Dental education, training and qualifications.

House surgeon Birmingham

I qualified in 1954 and my first job was house surgeon at the Birmingham Dental Hospital for six months. We used to rotate round, from the examination room, that is diagnostic and treatment planning, through to local anaesthetic department, through to the general anaesthetic department. I think we did periodontal attachments under the supervision of a chap called Dr Fox; we seemed to rotate around most of the departments except orthodontics.

I was paid 540 pounds for a year and, considering I'd earned nothing until then, I thought this was a jolly good start. The value of 540 was quite good in 1955.[10]

Then I did the second house surgeon's job, which was split between the dental hospital and the general hospital. That was a most interesting job because we were on duty every night of the week. There were two of us in this split job. We had a room in casualty, with no chair, just an operating bench where we did all our extractions and dressings. We used to use carbolised resin for toothache, because we didn't want to extract every tooth that came in because we'd get 50 or 60 people at a weekend. The demand was enormous. I mean really queues of people waiting. That was the second house job, which was far more formative, and we worked in theatre with a consultant on his operating lists. So here I was in the environment which I really wanted to be in.

The chief at the general hospital was R.W.H. Tavenner, who was doubly qualified, a very nice chap who was a single man – very unusual. He used to make us laugh because he said, 'I've got to go away for the weekend to see my aunt, could you look after the shop?' that was one of his statements, and the other one was, 'Oldham, keep a sticky eye on that,' meaning be very careful with what you were doing.

It wasn't terribly adventurous, the surgery was cysts, odontomas, extractions, a little bit of pre-prosthetic surgery, removing tuberosities if they were stopping a denture, anything like that, basic oral surgery really. If there was a malignant case, that was a big deal, a very big deal, and we got the plastic surgeons.

---

[10] £540 in 1955 was equivalent to £17,180 in 2022. In his resident oral surgery job at the Birmingham General Hospital, he would earn the same amount but accommodation and meals would be included.

Lawrence was called up for National Service in the Royal Air Force

We started in Blackpool at RAF Warton, then went down to RAF Halton for the second stage of training, two stages. We went through the six weeks induction. We were told about how the system works from a dental point of view because we were all going to be dental practitioners in the RAF.

We had to learn to march, and we were awful at it. The Dental Branch headquarters at Halton was in a Rothschild mansion where we all lived.[11] Each intake ended up at Halton. There was an ice rink which was surrounded by trees. We were so dreadful that we were made to march within the ice rink which had no ice in it; it was all concrete.

We got through the course and then it was the passing out night at Halton and everybody got absolutely inebriated. I can remember them coming down the stairs. There was a marvellous set of stair banisters, somehow sliding down on trays. And after about 11.30 I'd had enough of this so went up to my bedroom, which we shared as a dormitory, to find another dental graduate on his back vomiting and I thought, he'll get Mendelson syndrome unless I'm careful so I got him on his side and let the vomit out, because I'm sure he would have inhaled it, I mean he was way out. Anyway, it was my first resuscitative procedure.[12]

There were 12 in this intake, 12 aspiring dentists who'd joined the RAF. They said, 'Right, we're going to give you lots, you can draw the lots where you are going, they're all marked with the destination; they were sticks. I was the first to choose, and I drew out a stick which had on RAF Headquarters, London. And they were all terribly envious of this because they were all posted to Aden, Bahrain, Changi or Singapore or somewhere and I was going to be posted in London. So, the intake was spread all over the world because we still had bases in these places.

Harley Street

I pitched up at the RAF Headquarters in 114a Harley Street. In charge was Wing Commander Temple Tate, known as Dental Plate, Wing Commander Dental Plate. But he was a very nice man. He lived in Gerard's Cross and had a very nice uniform and he was a sort of benign uncle figure in the practice; he used to treat the air marshals, air vice

---

[11] Halton House and its estate was one of many owned by Alfred de Rothschild. It was purchased by the RAF on his death in 1918.

[12] Mendelson's syndrome: peptic-aspiration pneumonia, first described by Mendelson in 1946.

marshals, all the bigwigs on the ground floor in a very nice big surgery. Then upstairs I remember Geoffrey Forman, a very nice graduate from Guy's.[13] He ran a very successful practice on the first floor. I was upstairs on the third floor. The most exalted rank I ever got was squadron leaders; I mostly dealt with ranks below a squadron leader. I enjoyed it quite a lot. I was doing mainly amalgams and silicates, basic restorative work which I quite enjoyed, I took a pride in it, and remembered all my teaching.

Posting to Cambridge

I was posted to Cambridge and my world took on a totally new dimension because I was responsible for the dental surgery in a thousand-man station; we flew Vampire jets, and I was responsible for every aspect of dental surgery for all the staff, senior and junior and all the wives and families. It was a very good job and the first real practice job I'd taken on. Our dental surgery was part of the medical centre.

Dr Fanning was the squadron leader doctor in charge of the whole unit and I had a dental room and I took this over and really got it going. The first thing that happened was we had a parquet floor, and I set to and got this polished and raised the standard of the whole room so that it was shining beautifully for anybody who came in to have his dental treatment, it looked very clean and neat. I got known on the station for the cleanest dental place in the service. However, when we were inspected by a group captain who came from somewhere, he said, 'This is dangerous. Have you had anybody slip on this floor?' so whatever you did there was criticism. However, I thoroughly enjoyed the station, it was a happy life but restricted. I signed up to an external correspondence course for the primary and then I got able to use the medical school in Cambridge anatomy department library, because I was preparing for my primary.[14]

Dental Practice Wimpole Street

When I finished my National Service I went to Marylebone Library, looked at the British Dental Journal and found a vacancy in Wimpole Street. I applied to join the Wimpole Street practice and was interviewed and was accepted. I got references from the RAF and I was given the job in the basement. It didn't really suit me at all.

---

[13] Who became an oral and maxillofacial surgeon at King's College Hospital.
[14] Primary examination for the Fellowship in Dental Surgery of the Royal College of Surgeons of England.

I didn't do very well at all there, and in the end, I decided this wasn't for me and I would leave. It was a lot of crown and bridge which I wasn't good at, I did one crown in the air force, but that was it. By now I'd got this interest in surgery.

Upstairs was private and I remember the author Somerset Maugham going in to the first floor to be treated. We had quite a lot of hospital people. Many Bart's nurses came for treatment. I was like a fish out of water, really. When I threw in the towel, they got somebody from Australia to do it and he was much more aggressive and geared up to crown and bridge than I was.

Academic job in Manchester

I went to the British Dental Journal and there was a vacancy in Manchester, so I pitched up for an interview and was interviewed by Raddon, the professor who was an Australian. I think he got his chair because he'd done research in healing tooth extraction sockets.

Although he appointed me, I never gelled with him really, I felt he was always a little suspicious. He wasn't a chap you could easily relate to, not sure why. I started off in the dental anatomy teaching with Freddy Monks. Freddy Monks was the consultant at Bolton. He was a very good basic dental surgeon consultant who taught dental anatomy. I used to teach dental anatomy under him and then rotate from local anaesthesia clinics to general anaesthesia clinics.

I gradually improved and stayed there till 1965 which was five years. At the end of five years I was so bored and nothing was new I decided to do a masters. But the supervision was nil, and I picked a topic to do research on white lesions. I got no help from anybody. Now I can't understand why this was. I think in those days the university research wasn't geared and well organised at all, because I was left to flounder and not surprisingly, I made no progress at all and I thought, this is ridiculous, I'm just marking time, wasting. So, what with the tedium of repetitive teaching of successive year students, I thought, this is ridiculous, we'll take a few risks, and I applied to go to East Africa.

Laurence then went to the East Africa for two years and returned to oral surgery and eventually became a consultant in Taunton. His story continues in: The Making of British Oral and Maxillofacial Surgery. Sadler. A.

5. Oliver Gowers

Oliver started in commerce by selling rabbits in WWII and became employed in a warehouse of the Dental Manufacturing Company. He rose through the industry eventually starting Panadent introducing VITA vacuum fired and bonded porcelain to the domestic market. Oliver told his story of the evolution of the dental supply industry to Stephen Simmons at his home in 2012.

******

I was born in Croydon, Surrey, 1927. In the early days of the war, when I was 12, I was evacuated with two of my brothers to Hailsham in Sussex. Unfortunately we had a very low-level education, but we attended school in the mornings and visited the farms and other aspects in the afternoons. It was a very interesting life, but not good academically. After about nine months of being evacuated, I came home to Croydon but just in time for the Blitz to start. We experienced the bombing at Croydon airport and we all cycled over to see what we could see.

My beginnings were rather humble, and, at the age of 12, I started selling rabbits, this was the start of my selling career. My father built me four rabbit hutches and because of the war, meat was in short supply and my rabbits at one shilling and sixpence each were in quite healthy demand.

I left school at 14 and my father said I should go for an apprenticeship so I became an apprentice to a watch making firm in Croydon. But after about six or seven months, I found this didn't really suit my ambitions and so I looked around again, I thought I'd need something more technical, and I thought I'd become a dental technician.

So, my mother and I visited the DMC depot in Croydon, that's the Dental Manufacturing Company depot, because in those days they held a register of technicians and sometimes dentists looking for work opportunities. So I went into the DMC, they took me on until something came up as a dental technician, which didn't happen, I stayed with DMC for 24 years.

The Dental Manufacturing Company

In 1941 I was working in the depot and materials were very short because of the war, so the company looked for old stocks and, unfortunately, a lot of patients must have finished up with rather miscoloured teeth. But I came into the depot when new materials were progressing, although at the time we were selling rubber for vulcanites. Vulcanizers were messy, smelly things; we sold them to the dental laboratories. In those days, it was very common for dentists and dental technicians to visit depots to choose their requirements. And I spent a lot of time selecting teeth for dentists with their models. Platinum long pin teeth were popular, as were indeed slot facings and backings. And the very early tube teeth, which were mostly a lump of porcelain with a hole down the centre to fit a pin.

That type of thing was pretty amateurish, but it was showing signs of progressing all the time. And of course, so were the surgery products. We were selling, then, the first alginate. I remember I was very impressed. The material was Zelix, and that was selling for six shillings and six pence a tin. We sold loads of mercury for amalgam fillings and that was selling at nineteen shillings a pound, supplied in little porcelain jars.

There were others that came, SS White impression paste was quite popular. But Zelix had a problem with the trade name because they had to change it after a year or two from Zelix to Zalgan; and that was popular.

DMC in those days were popular manufacturers of dental equipment and dental materials. They were founded, I believe, in 1885 by a group of dentists who felt they could organise themselves into a company to supply and manufacture dental products. I can remember the early equipment such as the DMC 20th century chair, which had three cylinders. It was lower and higher than any other chair on the market and, although expensive, it was very popular.[15]

I also recall the Rathbone Unit, which was one of very few units on the market. Few dentists would afford to buy the German Ritter or Siemens equipment because it was too expensive. But DMC produced quite a vast range, as seen by their very early catalogues. Although I was

---

[15] See: The History of the Dental Manufacturing Company Ltd. Olivia Gambol. Dental Historian 2020 65 (1) 15-20.

quite young, I had an intimate knowledge of the products which ran into hundreds or thousands.

I used to have the job of cutting out gold plate, No 4 plate, for swaging. Dental laboratories were doing swaging at the time and cutting out gold clasps and that type of thing.

However, having worked at DMC for a few years I then joined the ATC, the Air Training Corps. I was with the ATC for about four years and then joined the RAF. I was selected for aircrew, but by this time, in 1945, the war was ending and I was re-mustered to join the Air Force as a storekeeper.

DMC were a good firm; they paid me whilst I was away in the RAF. When I went back to them after the war I was at the depot only a few months when the head office offered me a rise. They said that you can have a rise of five shillings if you stay here at DMC Croydon, or you can go to Glasgow. At the time I was eager to do different things so I went to Glasgow and spent two years as manager of the Glasgow depot, I was 22. That was good experience, I used to call on the Glasgow Dental Hospital and all the dentists' laboratories in Glasgow.

Dental salesman

Eventually I came back down to London, and DMC offered me a selling job on the road. I was given the opportunity to take over from one of their most experienced salesmen, Norman Pym. He was a very dapper sort of gentleman with his bowler hat. He was the last of the salesmen in London to be chauffeur driven around the West End and other parts of London. My job was mainly in Harley and Wimpole Streets and I did that for quite a time. I was disappointed with the equipment and state of affairs in Harley Street, in particular. I expected to find it all elaborate and modern, but indeed it was quite old-fashioned and not exceedingly good.

Then the company asked me to start a depot in Reading. It was 1951 or 1952. Materials were in very great demand and in very short supply because of the war and because of the extraordinary demand by the NHS coming into being. It was a crazy situation because the dental laboratories were receiving cases full of models and really couldn't cope with the work. Then the government, in their wisdom, decided then to put on a charge. Patients would pay a certain percentage of the cost and that, of course, reduced the demand considerably.

I had to search round Reading to find suitable premises and engage a small staff. We kept our own accounts and I had to purchase furniture, stock and everything else. In Reading the current salesman was unwell and getting ready for retirement, so I had to not only manage the depot but travel the areas in Surrey, Berkshire, Hampshire and part of Dorset.

After six years, the head office brought me back to London as their head office manager and after a short time, I was made retail sales manager. And then I was in charge of 13 dental depots around the country, and about 35 salesmen, so that kept me very busy. I had to visit all these salesmen and dental depots several times a year. And then, after a time, I felt I wanted my own business.

The start of Panadent

In the meantime, I was head hunted and joined the firm Truject, who had quite a good selection of products, mainly from Germany. I joined them as their managing director and I was there for three years. And then I was asked then to join the VITA Organisation, VITA Zahnfabrik of Germany, because I had quite a reasonable reputation at the time. I was invited to have their sole distributorship for the UK, which of course I took, gladly, and then started my own depot in London Road by the Elephant and Castle, South East London. That was the start of Panadent.

VITA, the start of vacuum fired porcelain and John McLean

As the VITA agent, I had the opportunity to progress porcelain and ceramics in general and had my first introduction to John McLean. During the first two years of distributing VITA, other German, Swiss, French and Italian firms wanted to join us. And after about two years we had about 20 agencies for the various manufacturers on the Continent.

I met John McLean and spent a lot of time with him at Panadent. We formed a small group to investigate the porcelain position because before then we were only using air fired porcelains which was fired at 680 degrees. There was then the possibilty of incorporating vacuum fired porcelains and this is where John McLean came into his own, so to speak.

He went to Germany to the VITA Organisation and spent a lot of time there experimenting with various porcelains. He eventually came back to London and we introduced the VITA vacuum fired teeth to the market and indeed the VITA vacuum furnace. John McLean was helped a lot in those days by a West End technician, Mick Cage, mainly, he was a very fine ceramist. And there were others in the area who did a good job in experimenting with vacuum fired porcelains because there was quite a lot of cracking and unfortunate colour deterioration in those days. That was overcome and the next project by John McLean was with bonded porcelain, this is bonding porcelain to metals. That was a big task

27

because of various problems, particularly with the cracking of teeth, discolouration and other problems. Eventually it was overcome and VITA introduced the bonded VMK porcelain. It became very popular and we were exceedingly busy at the time selling to all the dental laboratories throughout the UK. It was very successful.

John McLean was more than helpful in providing demonstrations and lectures and other helpful ideas about porcelain, discussing with various people throughout the country. And he was not to be put down by the German manufacturers or anyone else. He was very single-minded and certainly had a lot of opinions. But he was a very experienced man and did a lot of good for the dental technicians and dentists, and of course the patients who had the benefit of the work.

Of course, dentistry changed with the oncoming of the National Health. I well remember prior to National Health days it was a common thing for people to have all their teeth extracted and vulcanite or plastic dentures. Gradually various improvements in equipment and materials came onto the market.

DMC and the Wispair turbine drill

The biggest improvement, as far as I was concerned, was the air turbine drill. I went to the dental exhibition in Rome in 1960 and saw what I believe was the first turbine. It was most impressive, although very noisy and certainly a bit troublesome. And the firm DMC, which was run by two very experienced engineers, Frank and Percy Horton at their Blackpool factory, set about copying the turbine. They produced the DMC turbine which was known as the Wispair and that sold very well. And they also introduced the tungsten carbide bur, which was popular although very brittle and quite troublesome.

Training laboratory technicians

Having formed Panadent, my experience was quite extensive. And one of my ideas was to promote dental training and so we started a training laboratory at Panadent. We engaged Mr Dennison, who was a ceramist from Eastman Dental Hospital. He was our instructor and he did the teaching of these new VITA products, that's with vacuum formed porcelain and, latterly, of course, bonding of porcelain. We also engaged one of the best ceramists in London, Ian Potter, and he was very popular, and did a lot for us and the VITA organisation. But unfortunately, he died at a young age and his work had to be carried by other technicians, ceramists. So, we carried on with laboratories and today Panadent still has a main interest in teaching ceramists.[16] We do this mainly these days on a one-to-one basis, whereas previously we had courses for many ceramists.

In 1960 I became married to my wife Pat, and she was a great help in those days of establishing the firm, Panadent. She became company secretary and is still in that post and is still doing what she can to assist. When I was about 74, I retired and handed over the business to my son Peter, who had been with the firm for a number of years. He is now the managing director of Panadent and I am the Panadent Chairman.

Changes in the dental supply industry

Through my dental experiences I've seen a major change in dentistry. In the early days I had many visits to the dentists who were pulling out teeth galore and providing dentures. It's remarkable to see the improvements of today where you can see how people's teeth have very much improved. I'm glad to say that we had quite an influence over the provision of crowns and bridges.

The dentist today is a different type of character from the very early days before the NHS, when dentistry was on a different level. Dentists were always hard up but highly respected and today I'm glad to say that we have a great cooperation from the British Dental Association and other dental organisations.

One thing that comes to mind of course was the changing in the price situation because in the early days we had the retail price maintenance which was finished, I don't know exactly when, but probably in the 1950s. In those days we could be fined by our own association for selling at lower than recommended prices, whereas today of course it's all cut and thrust and bargains galore and price is of considerable interest. Of course, our company was always a member of the BDTA, the British Dental Trade Association, and we always did our best to assist wherever we could. I was on the council for quite several years and particularly at the onset of staff training and helped to produce the first training manual. In 1983 I became President of the Association and held the annual conference in Eastbourne.

One thing I think which interests people is how the dental trade decides what to stock and distribute. Because it's a big commercial decision and it has clinical implications and I think people often wonder

---

[16] He was speaking in 2012.

how do you make that decision? Do you have any discussion, clinical input from dentists or others? How do you decide things like that?

It can be quite a difficult decision in deciding what to introduce to the market because dental materials have always been expensive because of the relatively small number of items that can be produced. 30,000 dentists are a very small demand, really. And dentists and dental technicians are not willing to change products readily. They are very slow, particularly in Britain. In other places like Spain or Italy the dentists will change materials virtually overnight, which makes it easier for the dental suppliers. But introducing new products, which we've done of course many times, is a rather a slow process and one can make a big mistake of introducing materials too early on the market.

Fortunately, the dental supply industry has a close relationship with the dental schools and dental hospitals who are prepared to accept new materials for trial and testing. We had a very close relationship with the Eastman Dental Hospital, who tested our products and gave us reports on them which influenced us to either to go ahead with production or dismiss it. And indeed, a lot of dentists have new ideas and put new ideas to dental suppliers, but they may not be economically viable simply because the demand is not appropriate for that product. It might only sell a few dozen or something, which is not enough for a production run.

But companies like DMC at the time had a thriving factory at Blackpool, where I worked for some time, producing and experimenting with products. Many of them never came onto the market but others did and were very successful. We had cooperation from various dentists and dental laboratories throughout the country to do testing for us and reporting. Of course, eventually one needs a dentist to provide instruction, as indeed when we introduced an implant product, we had to find a dentist who could carry out instruction work. One needs that type of cooperation from the profession to promote one's products.

6. *Professor Sir Paul Bramley*

Paul Bramley studied dentistry during WWII and later medicine. After volunteering in Africa as a medical missionary he trained in oral surgery and spent 16 years as a consultant in Plymouth before becoming a professor and subsequently Dean at the Sheffield dental school. He spoke about anaesthesia which was a particular interest, practically, educationally and politically. He also spoke about being on the General Dental Council, chair of Dental Protection and Dean of the Faculty of Dental Surgery of the Royal College of Surgeons of England. I interviewed Sir Paul at his home over two days in 2014.

******

Being a dental Student in Birmingham during WWII

Most of the college wanted to go into medicine, but I didn't think of myself in those terms, so I went into dentistry. It was partly because my mother took me to a very distinguished dental practice where both partners were doubly qualified. And I was influenced by one of my contacts, a person about 10 or 15 years older me, also a young dentist in Leicester. I thought that's a good life, that's what I'll do.

I decided I would get qualified in dentistry and practise dentistry but with a medical qualification. It was the glamour of this practice in Leicester and their insistence to my mother than really dentistry is all right but you'd be better off if you were medically qualified as well.

I signed up for Birmingham. I didn't like the sound of Guy's, so I went to Birmingham. The way that dental hospitals were run before the advent of full-time academic teachers, was the honorary consultant system. That meant they gave their services to Guy's, Bart's, the London Hospital, etc, for free, but you got the student contact for future referrals, got the kudos of working at a great teaching hospital. You also had your private practice in Wimpole Street or Harley Street or thereabouts, which flourished under this and financed your largesse in teaching in a dental hospital. That was the payoff. In Birmingham they were distinguished, local people who came into the dental hospital perhaps once or twice a week, and retired back to their own practices.

As an undergraduate dental student, you went into the GA department and you did half the anaesthetics or half the extractions that morning until 11 o'clock. From 9 to 11, you were at it all the time. So, you had a huge soaking in nitrous oxide and oxygen, there wasn't any Trilene then, and some brute force.

It was wartime, and I lived in the old VD[17] ward in the general hospital in Birmingham, which was absolutely the centre of Birmingham, next door to all the industrial installations and it was a pretty dangerous place. But we fire watched there for one shilling a night, and a bed-and-breakfast and an evening meal in the general hospital, Steelhouse Lane.[18]

When we had air raids and incendiary bombs, you had to get up on the roof and deal with them, which we did on several nights, and that was pretty scary because the firemen were coming up with their hosepipes, not seeing you on the roof, and these great jets of water came round.

During that time, the Birmingham General Hospital had the biggest casualty outpatients in Europe; there was a huge turnover in central Birmingham, particularly in wartime. We used to man casualty in the evenings, if we'd got nothing better to do, I was the one dental student; the other ten or eleven people were medical students. We bailed out of our wards into casualty and I got all the anaesthetics to do because, unlike the medical students, I had some knowledge of suffocation and the problems. I got a lot of practical hands-on things to do as well as the dental hospital stuff. Anaesthetics were just part of dentistry.

After dental school, a dental house job in Birmingham and National Service in the far east Paul Bramley returned to Birmingham to study medicine. But he needed to earn a living.

Part-time dental practice as a medical student

I went into dental practice. It was then 1948. In 1948, the Health Service started, and it was very easy to get patients. I found, through a girlfriend, that her father had died about 12 years before and had run a practice on Hagley Road in Birmingham, a good address. But nobody had taken it on; they didn't sell it, it just was there, and vacant. And I said that I was thinking of starting in practice and wondered if her mother would be interested. So I was invited to see her.

---

[17] Venereal disease.

[18] The Birmingham General Hospital in Steelhouse Lane closed in the 1990s and is now the Birmingham Children's Hospital

There was this ancient Ritter unit – which was the thing to have 20 years before – an ancient chair, carpet on the floor, a mahogany thing with pull-out drawers that all the instruments were in, and a boiling water steriliser. And what's more, a very matronly person, dressed in a classic maid's gown, was there. She had been his old chair-side assistant, and she was looking after the family. So I went into there.

One of my medical student colleagues had done dental assisting in the RAMC.[19] He was interested in earning a bit, so he assisted me. So two medical students attended two evenings a week and weekends. We went over on a motorbike and got going with this.

I had no problems. I moved about in a circle of people whom I had qualified with as a dentist, who were doctors, who were now teaching us as new medical students. A lot of the staff came over and we had a very distinguished clientele, which I treated on the Health Service. What the quality of the work was, I really don't know. I did the best I could.

So that put me in a position then to enjoy a big social life because of all the contacts I'd had in two generations. Evening and weekend practice gave me enough to buy a really ancient Ford 8, which eventually I had to back up the hills because the fourth gear wouldn't work the right way round. And have a foreign holiday. And what's more, I found out much later in life that my years in that practice counted towards my entitlement of the years served in the NHS for my pension, a wonderful present to have.

Sir Paul became an oral and maxillofacial surgeon in Plymouth for 16 years and subsequently Professor at the dental school in Sheffield. He spent some time as the Dean and sat on the General Dental Council.

I sat on the General Dental Council as the representative of the University of Sheffield, it was not to do with the deanship. I really don't know how I was appointed.

My relationships with the General Dental Council were not good. Its President had been Bradlaw[20] for several years. Hindley-Smith was the Registrar when I first went there and he was a very good man. He was dignified, he knew his way about the Privy Council and gave wonderful

---

[19] Royal Army Medical Corps.
[20] Sir Robert Bradlaw. Dean of the Newcastle Dental School and later of the Eastman Dental Institute, Chair of the General Dental Council, First Dean of the Faculty of Dental Surgery of the Royal College of Surgeons of England, Present of the British Dental Association. Plarr's Lives of the Fellow. Royal College of Surgeons, available online.

dinners. The General Dental Council dinner was the dinner that people in the London circuit wanted to get onto. The wines were superb, the cook was great and they were marvellous occasions. I do recognise that as being a high point in my culinary life.

It was a well-run organisation, quietly run, but I didn't like the way they appointed new Presidents. It was all done by the machinations of Hindley-Smith and a few of the elder statesmen who presented you with a person to be elected. Someone made a speech of proposal and there was never any opposition.[21]

The centre of it was its President who was conservative to the nth degree and didn't want change. In fact, I know they didn't want change because it was retold to me back that when I was Dean of the London Faculty,[22] both Lawton[23] and his new Registrar, who was Davis, a man I liked well, an ex-artillery colonel, I think. And the President was thinking about his succession. And Lawton turned to Davis. He said, 'Bramley's an innovator and we don't want that, do we?' So that was my death knell regarding him.

He tried to say I couldn't possibly be a council member of the Medical Protection Society and serve on the General Dental Council. I said, 'Are you telling me, Frank, that I don't know how to behave, that I would let any vested interest go either way? I refute that entirely and I'm going to continue on both bodies as far as I feel myself accepted. So shut up about that.' But our relationship from then onwards was rather acid. What I didn't like, it was all 'keep it quiet', play by what the Privy Council wanted us to do, you're a subset of them and don't rock the boat, and enjoy your dinners. So I couldn't be doing with a lot of this.

I was given a chance to chair one of the disciplinary committees when someone was away. But anyway, I was persona non grata, absolutely, and I didn't like their ways of shutting up general discussion.

It was an atmosphere which I really can't comment on positively and it seems to me, if I look at what the British Dental Association is up to, I can't comment positively on them either in their present form.[24]

---

[21] See: David Dury Hindley-Smith (1916-2001), The Dental Board of the UK and the General Dental Council. Gelbier S. Dental Historian 2022 67(1).
[22] Faculty of Dental Surgery of the Royal College of Surgeons of England.
[23] Sir Frank Lawton was Director of Dental Education at the Liverpool Dental School and became President of the General Dental Council and British Dental Association.
[24] He was speaking in 2014.

Council member of the Medical Protection Society

As a Council member, I attended the Council meetings, which were once every two months or something like that. They were mostly case committees, 'Should we defend, shouldn't we?' that sort of thing.

There was the retirement of the senior dentist who was dealing with dental matters in the Society, and we appointed David Phillips. He was a dentist in South Wales, Bristol graduate, very successful, very active in local politics. Between us, we arranged to form Dental Protection as a subgroup and we ran our own affairs.[25] And I then became Chairman of Dental Protection and I did that for six years after I had retired, until I was 72.

I did a big analysis of the sort of cases we had to deal with, as part of my offering as chairman. I went through things and found out what were the flavours of the months. But the sort of things were accidents in practice, fractured mandible after use of elevators under local, which they should never have been done without bone removal, that sort of thing; were we going to defend or were we not? Taking out the wrong teeth, molesting women patients. There was quite a lot of stuff really which emanated from a failure to recognise that something had gone wrong and to apologise to the patient and not coming clean. And all that had increased.

We were defending people in the General Dental Council, that's why I was thought to have been a problem by being on council of both organisations. So it was all sorts of miscreants, Geoffrey Howe was one, he was a client, with this Hong Kong business.[26] There was a whole spectrum of miscreants who had done things like fiddling their books and defending people who had had a criminal conviction.

---

[25] Dental Protection Limited became a separate company within the Medical Protection Society in 1989.

[26] Geoffrey Howe was the first professor of oral surgery in the UK. Initially in Newcastle and subsequently at the Royal Dental Hospital. He was a gifted teacher and dental politician. He designed the dental school in Hong Kong and subsequently became the first Dean. But there was a scandal concerning the supply of equipment for the new hospital by a company involving his wife. He lost the job in Hong Kong and became a professor in Jordan. His memoir 'Reflections of a Fortunate Fellow' is in the British Dental Association library and there are some available through Amazon.

Council member of the Faculty of Dental Surgery of the Royal College of Surgeons of England

I was Dean from 1980 to 1983. I'd served on the Board of Faculty and of the Council of the College before I was Dean, for quite a time, so I knew what was going on and I had seen the style of various Deans.

The faculty is all about professional standards, it's supposed to have nothing to do, in those days, with politics. That it must impinge on politics is neither here nor there. You were supposed to be careful of that. I felt that who was chosen as Dean, every three years, reflected what the faculty thought of the last Dean and what was required in the next Dean.

So you got people like Hovell who was a maniacal Dean.[27] You never knew what he was going to do, great enthusiast and personality.

But there were one or two public disasters, it needed somebody to settle the ship down. Who did they elect? Ken Lindow, who was the prosthetics professor at King's, but he was a kind, steady, gentle man who dealt well with people, not the flair, but some of the drive and direction that Hovell had. But he hadn't got the edge of the volcano feeling you had every time John Hovell stood up in public. What was going to happen? But they settled on that sort of chap and it was that sort of regime.

When I came on board, I felt there was a need for radical action. The faculty was merely responding to outside events. The government would put a paper before us about changes, the British Dental Association would produce something, some outside agency would say, 'What do you think about this?' and we will respond.

I said that we needed to think about the basic problems ourselves and get organised and researched in such a way that we have faculty attitudes to some of the major problems before we get asked for them. We've had to lead this. So I went to Johnson Gilbert, who was Secretary of the College, and said, 'Look, I'm not going to try to make a new qualification or have ideas about changing the structure of the faculty or anything like that. My intention is to leave this faculty a more thinking organisation

---

[27] John Hovell was a consultant at the Royal Dental Hospital where he practiced orthodontics and at St Thomas's Hospital where he was an oral surgeon. He had a reputation for innovation in major oral and maxillofacial surgery. See: John Herbert Hovell (1910-1988), TD, MRCS, LRCP, FRCS, FDSRCS (Eng.), FFD (Ire), D Orth. Gelbier S. Journal of Medical Biography 2016 May; 24(2); 145-57.

than it is today. That certainly needs to be done, and it's a big job, and this is how I'm going to do it.' So he eventually approved.

But we had, 'What about the faculty and general dental practice? Do we have a responsibility over and above them having one LDS representative on the Board? What's going to happen if we do nothing about this?' I thought we should get a sub-committee of our mates from within the Board and get on and look at the implications of our relationship with the general practice of dentistry.

There were other topics; one was the examination system, particularly the fellowship examination system, to look at that yet again.

Dominance of Oral Surgery in Faculty of Dental Surgery

In Bradlaw's mind, when he set up the faculty, he set up the Fellowship and he thought this should be an exam to encourage dentists to behave and be capable of acting as the consultant dental surgeons in the hospital environment. So it was medicine and surgery orientated.

Of course, the people who took that exam were doing what was probably, but not then known as, oral surgery. It was probably still dental surgery, but they were doing oral surgery insofar as it was. They were the majority, and they picked up the votes because they were the people who were known, who had got their FDS and they were qualified to do it, and they clung onto that, against all the orthodontists and so on. [28]

I felt, probably because of our thinking expedition, that we ought to be wider based if we were going to survive as a faculty. We should include general practice, the orthodontists and all the other specialities, get them a place on the Board so they could speak for the width of dentistry from an academic point of view.

Paul Bramley had been taught to give anaesthetics as a dental student in Birmingham. He became the dental house surgeon at the Queen Elizabeth Hospital in Birmingham.

---

[28] The first Fellowships in Dental Surgery were granted by examination at the Royal College of Surgeons of England in 1948, soon after the Faculty of Dental Surgery was formed in 1947, and in Edinburgh in 1949. The first candidates to pass were: Norman Rowe, Homer Killey and Tom Battersby, seven candidates took the exam. See: Gelbier S. 125 years of developments in dentistry, 1880–2005. Part 5: Dental education, training and qualifications. British Dental Journal, 199 (2005) 10 685 - 689. *And:* The Faculty of Dental Surgery of the Royal College of Surgeons of England: An overview of the first 70 years of achievements. Stephens C. Dental Historian 2017; 62(1) 24 - 32.

When I was dental house surgeon to Harold Round,[29] his partner in his Birmingham practice was a woman called Jessie Rowbotham, who was a foil for the great man. She used to have to do the dental extractions at this Monyhull Colony[30] and she asked me to give her anaesthetics. So without being appointed and so on, I used to turn up to her clinics when she did extractions and I did the anaesthesia. It was all very informal, that's what life was like then.

What did I give? It was plain, straightforward nitrous oxide and plenty of oxygen, a lot of skill and occasionally squirts of ethyl chloride onto a pack when people got really stroppy. By the time I came to Monyhull Colony, I was pretty experienced in dental anaesthesia and did a far better job of it than the general practitioners who used to give anaesthetics for dentists.

Also, I used to give anaesthetics for the ENT list in the Queen Elizabeth Hospital as the dental house surgeon, and that was Schimmelbusch mask, and pour on the ether for all their quickies. Why I was doing it and the department of anaesthetics not doing it, I really don't know. It all happened like this. It was very casual.

When I started in dental practice myself during medical qualification, there were two cylinders on the floor, one of nitrous oxide and one of oxygen, and you stood on them and turned the taps on and off with your foot and gave the anaesthetic through a nose mask and that was straight forward nitrous oxide/oxygen. But once I frightened myself stiff by giving a general anaesthetic and doing an extraction at the same time, and the chap stopped breathing. But we got him round in the end and he was all right.

Anaesthesia as Professor of Oral Surgery at the Sheffield Dental School.

I really had my trouble later on as Professor of Oral Surgery. The General Dental Council specified what you had to do about dentists giving general anaesthetics and what practical work they had to do. The

---

[29] Harold Round had qualified as a dentist in Birmingham in 1906. He was one of the first two dentists in Britain to qualify with a BDS degree in dentistry, the other was John Whittles. Previously dentists had qualified with an LDS diploma from one of the Royal Colleges, had a medical qualification or no qualification at all. See: 125 years of developments in dentistry, 1880–2005 Part 5: Dental education, training and qualifications. Gelbier S. British Dental Journal 199 (2005) 685–688.

[30] The Monyhull Colony was a mental hospital at King's Norton near Birmingham. It was a self-sufficient community with the patients working the farmland to supply their own needs.

Professor of Anaesthetics had a very different view, and I had an absolute stand-up row in which he became livid and lost his temper and I finished by trembling myself. It got to that pitch.

I had a duty to do and was bloody well going to do it, and he felt he had a duty to mankind. It was all in the early days of the intravenous stuff with Drummond-Jackson,[31] so that stirred up the anaesthetic community. I had to teach it so it was a very uncomfortable time with the Professor. I think he had done his stuff at Guy's and scared himself when he trained, scared himself stiff with dental anaesthetics and really wanted a tube down for every one of them, which is ridiculous.

Paul Bramley was a member of the working parties for the Wyllie and Seward reports into general anaesthesia in dentistry. He tried to get a compromise in Sheffield.

I tried to sell a compromise but I don't think the anaesthetists bought it. But they assented to it and that was first to decide what dental anaesthesia was and secondly what training was needed. This was used politically as a get out by the anaesthetists, knowing probably full well we would never get that training. However, some people did a house officer's full general anaesthetic attachment in the major general anaesthetic department. But that scheme never really got to first base. The politics at that time was pretty difficult.

The Drummond-Jackson legal case

There was the case with Drummond-Jackson in the British Medical Journal, and Robinson in Birmingham, one of the longest libel cases there has ever been.

Drummond-Jackson was a dentist who lived in Sheffield, who was very good to us when we came as strangers. But he ran this West End practice, and he came into prominence with Brietal, methohexitone, short-term intravenous anaesthesia just a breath away from full consciousness. There had been one or two unfortunate deaths in anaesthesia, as there always are, whatever sort it is and whoever gives it. But it was being pinned by the anaesthetists on dental anaesthesia.

Drummond-Jackson's method was tested by Professor Robinson in Birmingham, the Professor of Anaesthesia there, who published a paper, which showed that they were doing dangerous things with methohexitone, physiologically, and the level of anaesthesia they were

---

[31] More tales of Stanley Drummond-Jackson see chapters 11 & 12.

achieving.[32] Drummond-Jackson, in reading the paper, went berserk because it was his method, and so he went about trying to get some of the research papers, workup papers and so on.

He found out they had not used Drummond-Jackson's method, but they had stressed Drummond-Jackson's method to an extent that it was dangerous. And that was the core of the thing, that the BMJ had published and making out that Drummond-Jackson's method was dud.

Drummond-Jackson case was that it wasn't his technique; it had been over-stressing to get their required results. And they argued for 18 months in front of the Judge, all sorts of people appeared. The Judge was very skilled in anaesthetic techniques by the time he'd finished with that lot, all the opinions that were given. And finally, he said, 'Come on, chaps, this is the longest case there's ever been in a libel case like this. We're getting nowhere. I suggest the costs have got right out of hand on both sides. You'd better call it a day.' So they called it off.

One day I got a telephone call when I was in theatre and I came out between cases. It was Eli Lilly.[33] They said they were going to run a joint meeting on dental and obstetric anaesthesia in relation to Brietal at the posh hotel opposite Harrods's. They wanted me to chair the meeting. The Society for the Advancement of Anaesthesia in Dentistry and Professor Robinson's group from Birmingham would be there. I thought this sounded like a sticky wicket.

So I went. Drummond-Jackson's gang and Robinson's all came along and I knew from seeing how they were sitting, my only function would be to intercepting pots. It was that sort of meeting. And they battled backwards and forwards and we got absolutely nowhere with it. They just insulted one another.

But I was on Drummond-Jackson's side, but wanting to temper his enthusiasms and it evolved into other stuff, resuscitation teaching and that sort of thing.

Sir Paul also talked about his career as an Oral and Maxillofacial Surgeon. See: The Making of British Oral and Maxillofacial Surgery. Sadler. A.

---

[32] Wise C, Robinson J, Heath M, Tomlin, P. British Medical Journal 1969 2; 540–543.
[33] Manufactures of Brietal, trade name of methohexitone.

7. Alan Seaton

Alan qualified from Manchester in the 1950s and initially worked in the Schools' Dental Service in deprived Oldham before buying a practice. Later he also worked as a dentist for Shell chemicals and, after becoming bored and disillusioned, he worked for the Dental Estimate Board and later Dental Protection. Alan was interviewed at the British Dental Association headquarters by Ros Levenson in 2014.

******

I was born in Altrincham in Cheshire in 1936; my father was a dentist in Manchester. We were evacuated to Mobberley in Cheshire during the war, and came back to live in the family house in Moss Side in Manchester, which was at that stage a relatively genteel area. I went to Manchester Grammar School and Manchester University qualifying in December 1960. I lived at home while I was studying.

It was rather expected that I would do dentistry. My father and his brother were dentists and they were both on the same page of the 1936 Dental Register. It was an expectation I followed. There was no career guidance that I can recall at school. It was expected that if you went into the science sixth biology department you were going to do medicine or an allied trade. I found a photograph of my year in the Sixth Form, and all those names I could remember, a vast preponderance of them having either done medicine or dentistry. So, it was a path that I followed.

A change in the dental course

I started dental school in September 1955. In those days, it was a five-year and one term course because we did the first MB/BDS year. We all thought it was to get money for the botany, zoology and physics department; we had to do what was the equivalent of A-Levels, which we'd already done. That took the first year. If you were very good at your A-Levels, you could skip the first year, but I wasn't very good at my A-Levels. But it was a very pleasurable time.

The lecturers and tutors varied; some were extraordinarily helpful. I suffered to some extent because my father, being a dentist in Manchester, knew some of them; I tried, if possible, to stay away from the people that he knew. Some of them were fine, but others were very high handed. But in the main the teaching that we had was first class.

The first two years consisted mainly of lectures, and then we became apprentice technicians and we spent a year in a place called junior lab, where we made dentures from start to finish.

Later we were let loose on patients with teeth, but only after we had done another couple of terms where we filled teeth in weird looking phantom heads, and then we were let loose on the public. We also did what nowadays I think is called minor oral surgery, but in our day, it was called local extractions. Manchester was a port and we would have frequent shiploads of crews who would come up and sit outside the dental hospital in lines. Those spitting blood you knew had been seen, and the others were waiting to be seen. We were looked upon as a clinic for the docks and we saw vast numbers of patients.

We had lots of experience. One particular teacher was a very nice chap called Ted Seeley, and for the first tooth I ever extracted he held my hand to make sure that I actually got the specific movements correct. I think I must have washed my hands about six times before I actually grasped hold of the forceps and removed the tooth. We didn't wear gloves. I don't remember which tooth it was, but I do remember the hand washing as some sort of delaying the dreadful moment you're actually pulling the tooth out. I was a little nervous.

Then we were given a list of patients and we had to see them and sort out exactly what their problems were, in different categories. We were given denture and conservation patients of our own, and we had to take them through all the way, each stage being checked by a lecturer. Some lecturers one avoided, one in particular because he was very fussy. We had to get everything signed for, and one of my colleagues became an expert forger. We learnt general anaesthetics; orthodontics was a very poor course and oral surgery was not something that you did as a student.

And then it all culminated in taking your final exam. The written bits of the exams were not as hard as they might appear, because there was only a limited number of questions and one used to trawl through previous papers, which were freely available. The practical part was something which by then had become just routine, really.

By then we had been five and a half years, and I think people were fed up of being students by that stage. It was good in the first three years, because you knew so many people, but then they'd all graduated and you had lost them, so it was a bit boring towards the end.

We qualified the week after National Service finished. National Service finished, I think, on December the 6th, and we qualified round about the 12th. We'd all been for medicals and one chap was called up. So, we missed National Service, which I regret in some respects.[34]

One chap was held back for a year and actually didn't take his finals. Another girl failed, which surprised everybody, her father was a dentist, but everybody else passed. We didn't have distinctions or honours or anything like that, you either passed or failed.

I would think we were a small year, maybe 25, and there were seven or eight girls, which I think was quite rare in those days. Two of them qualified and got married and I don't think ever did any dentistry. They'd wasted five and a half years; it seemed a pity.

The social life was extraordinarily good. It was at a time when Manchester University was big, but not as big as it is now, and there were always good relationships. If you went into town, everybody wore scarves, as some sort of badge, I suppose. And you were treated with respect, which I suspect might have gone nowadays. The Students' Union was an old building which they demolished and started again, and that was where we used to congregate on the Saturday night. I had a friend who had a trombone and played in a jazz band, and we used to go together to his gigs, and he would carry the case and I'd carry the trombone, or vice versa, and we'd both get in for nothing. So, it was a jolly time. We didn't behave badly.

There were no university fees. I had a grant which was £14 a term. Why that came about, I don't know, but obviously it was based on your parents' finances. The guy with the trombone had a full grant for all his time at university. When he started his father was a solicitor's clerk and he was between jobs and technically unemployed, and nobody ever asked him again for the following five years. But I was well supported by my parents and I was very lucky in that respect.

My father was always interested in my studies. He was in the first War and he must have qualified in the late 1920s. And things really hadn't moved on between the late 1920s and the 1950s in real terms, so he was

---

[34] The National Service act was passed in 1947 to keep military manpower available after WWII for continuing British commitments, particularly in Germany, Palestine, and India. It came into force in 1949 and all fit young men had to serve in the armed forces for 18 months which was extended to two years during the Korean war. Students and apprentices could defer until they had finished their studies. It ended in 1960.

always very interested in what was going on. And because of his association with committees, he knew quite a lot of the teachers, which was a disadvantage in some respects.

I think the teaching we had imbued us with the idea that dentistry was a bit more than blood and sawdust, and the teachers were generally more skilful than the dentists in practice. Some of them were part-timers, but they all had what appeared to be a very much a better view of dentistry than dentists at large.

Of course, there were still a lot of registered dentists about in those days who were unqualified but came onto the register in the Dentists' Act of 1922. [35] Some of them had been technicians, or mechanics as they were known in those days, who had drifted into dentistry as much as anything else. And they didn't have any real skills, in conservative dentistry, by and large. They were extraction and denture people.

School dental service

After qualification I tried to join a practice. There was a new surgery being built but at the time there was a huge backlog and nobody could get dental equipment. So, for the time being I worked in the School Service, which I think is now called the Community Service, it was Schools entirely in those days in Oldham. It was an eye opener. It mostly involved traipsing around schools, anaesthetising kids, and extracting vast numbers of decayed teeth.

---

[35] The first dentists' register was compiled after the 1878 Dentists' Act. It was held and administered by the General Medical Council. From August 1st 1879 the act forbade the use of the title dentist, dental practitioner or any title implying registration from anyone not registered. To be registered you had to be qualified with an LDS diploma, a medical qualification or prove you were already practicing dentistry. It didn't stop unregistered people from practicing. This led to the formation of the Society of Extractors and Adaptors of Teeth to represent the interests of unregistered practitioners.
The dentist act 1922 amended the previous act. Dentistry could only be practiced by registered persons or those with a medical qualification. A chemist or druggist could remove teeth in an urgent situation if no dentist was available provided no anaesthetic was used. To be registered you had to be qualified or have practiced dentistry for five of the previous seven years, been a member of the Incorporated Dental Society or been a dental mechanic for five of the previous seven years. Once registered you could call yourself dentist.
See: 125 years of developments in dentistry, 1880–2005 Part 2: Law and the dental profession Gelbier. S British Dental Journal, 199 (2005) 470–473. Also: Dentist Act 1878 and 1922 sourced in British Dental Association library.

The dental health of those children was very poor, and Oldham was a fairly deprived area. I did a bit of routine conservation, but by and large the parents didn't want it. Not for financial reasons, I think just historically they weren't used to having anything. It was not uncommon, in the north, for the 21st birthday present to a daughter to have all her teeth out and dentures. Now I was of the generation who wouldn't do it, whereas the previous generation, I think, had done it because traditionally that's what was done.

I enjoyed that part of my career for a while, and then it became really quite boring, just toddling out and gassing all these kids. You'd have queues of maybe 10 or 15. The bigger schools would have their own little dental surgery and we would take instruments with us.

The anaesthetist was usually a local GP who had an interest in anaesthetics; not necessarily any skill in it, but an interest. And you got them on the dusky side of pink. In other words, anoxic as near as dammit, and then you could dive in. But you only had a limited length of time, probably less than five minutes, to carry out any extractions.

I think the skills were very different from what they are now. Conservative treatment was not popular. The drills were bone shakers. They would do maybe 600 or 700 revolutions a minute, with luck. The air rotor came in in about 1959, I think. I never used one as a student. They went up to several hundred thousand rpm., so there was no, or very much less, vibration. You got a good smell of burning now and again, as we didn't cool things down. So conservative dentistry in those days, with slow drills, was jolly hard going both for the patient and the dentist, and I would imagine the high-speed drill cut down preparation time by a good 80 percent. Local anaesthetics improved, although they were pretty good in those days, anyway. So, it was what there was available at the time. That was the way you went about things in those days.[36]

After the School Dentistry Service, I started work in a practice. The practice finally got the equipment, and I was able to start work there. It was entirely Health Service. It was early 1961.

---

[36] Work started on the development of an air turbine in the 1940s but further developments continued in the 1950s to produce a commercially viable instrument See: The Origins of the Air-turbine Dental Handpiece. C Cherry, M Gibbons J & Ronayne. British Dental Journal. 136. (1974) 469–472.

Dental practice and living over the shop

I moved to Macclesfield, where I worked with a chap with whom I'd been at school. His father also was a dentist, and knew my father. The idea was that I would go there and eventually there would be a partnership offered, but the partnership kept being put off. This was a common problem with people of my generation. They would be encouraged to go into a practice on the basis that, 'after a couple of years we'll see about a partnership,' and that rarely materialised. I certainly know three or four other people who had exactly the same experience as me. We never fell out, it just kept being, 'Well, leave it another six months.' So, I decided I wanted to get out, and that was when I moved to South Manchester where I bought a practice.

By then of course everybody had air rotors, and work was more related to conservative treatment. We used to have a GA session once a week, but there were no more the troops of people coming through. It had become slightly less brutal by then.

I was working alone, but with a receptionist and a nurse. It was a cottage industry; the surgery and waiting room were on the ground floor. There had been a laboratory in the cellar, but that wasn't used. And I was living upstairs, which was quite normal at that time. I lived above the shop for four years. I was married by then, with a son and a daughter, who was born there.

It was a good community, a good, solid, middle-class clientele. They were all workers. They all usually owned their own houses and were nice folk to work with. We had a good oral surgery department in the local hospital, half a mile away. I had an anaesthetist who was a proper anaesthetist, not a GP masquerading as an anaesthetist, and he worked in the hospital. So, I had a contact there to refer patients to the hospital. I didn't refer a lot, and occasionally would refer people into the dental hospital. But I managed just about everything really.

Patients' charges for National Health Service treatment

Initially, the patient's contribution to treatment was £1.50 for everything. Then they introduced a percentage of the fees as a payment. And then in 1975, the National Health Service dropped the exempt age from 21 to 16, unless in full-time education and that did not mean going to university, that meant being at school. And at that stage, the patient's contributions became a great deal more significant, and not unnaturally patients were put off. There was a habit at one time of the 21-year-old barrier. People would say, 'Oh, I can't be bothered, but I know next year

I'm going to have to pay, so I'd better get my treatment done,' and that changed things quite dramatically. 1973 to 1975 was, I particularly recall, a good year financially. And then in 1975, there was enormous inflation which rather put the kibosh on that.

Too much treatment

Patients, generally speaking, came every six months. That was the norm at the time, and oral hygiene was pretty grim, so there was quite a lot of work to do. And, of course, dentistry begets dentistry. What I mean is that there was a temptation at one time to do too much treatment, and that treatment breaks down eventually, and then the treatment becomes more radical. I've been to the dentist once in the last 30 something years. So, as I've got older, the more I realise people should stay away from dentists, not go to them. That doesn't go down terribly well, I'm afraid.

I didn't have a hygienist; there were not hygienists that I can recall, certainly at that time. I was trying to educate patients about oral hygiene. But by and large you were pushing at a closed door. You did your best, and it seemed to have no effect whatsoever.

There was a great deal of opposition to fluoridation. Our water came from the Lake District, so presumably it would have been Manchester Corporation at one time, and they, I don't think, ever got involved in fluoridation. There were tests when South and North Shields was the area where they fluoridated North Shields water supply, but not South Shields. And that was quite a clever scheme and had some very good results.

Out of hours toothache and Saturday work

I was in the phonebook. There was no restriction for anybody calling. I used to work five and a half days a week, including Saturday morning, until people started fading. I remember I had a family due in on a Saturday morning, and they didn't turn up. And I saw them over the road, going into a shop, and I thought right, that's it, I'll give up Saturday mornings. That was the late 1960s. But if people called me out of hours, I would come downstairs and see them.

I stayed there until July 1985. In the meantime, I'd had an assistant or associate working with me. I had been offered a role in the local chemical works, which didn't sound brilliant, but it was Shell Chemicals and they had a very good dental setup. I was asked if I would go there. I think it was two half days a week, which I was happy to do.

Dental surgeon to Shell Chemicals

There had been a dental officer there, and he had left. It was very different from the practice. The physical setup was absolutely first class. Shell Chemicals was on the crest of a wave at the time and seemed to have money coming out of its ears, so if you wanted anything at all, you immediately got it. Dentistry is a very lonely job, by and large, but in this clinic, there was the medical officer, an optician, physiotherapist, assorted nurses. It was much more of a community job, which I enjoyed being part of. There were other people there to speak to, whereas in practice there's nobody to speak to at all because you're working all the time. You speak to patients, but you get a little fed up with that after a while.

It was mainly conservative dentistry, all Health Service stuff. There was no suggestion that Shell paid for the treatment. It was a nice experience. The equipment and facilities were slightly better than what I had at my practice. The whole place had been re-equipped about a year before I went. And there were two of everything and three of most things, and the equipment itself was very up to date.

Oral Hygiene

I used to find that the people working at Shell had a higher standard of oral hygiene. They seemed to be more aware of things. But I still realised that by the time I got back to the surgery, I was still in the same old problem of an inability to persuade people to do anything with their teeth.

I always remember one particular lovely lady. She was a school dinner lady. And she had the filthiest mouth you have ever seen in your entire life. And every six months she'd come in and I'd clean her up, and I'd say, 'You really must do something about it. You know, we'll give you a toothbrush.' If she had a toothbrush, she certainly never used it. And I could have seen that woman every three weeks and it wouldn't have made the slightest difference. She was a charming lady, but she didn't care. Well, that didn't happen at Shell Chemicals.

Disenchantment with dental practice

I carried on with this until 1985, and then I applied to join the Scottish Dental Estimates Board as a dental advisor. I didn't get the job because, quite rightly, I had no knowledge of the Scottish scene. And then I applied for the same role at the England and Wales Dental Estimates Board, which was in Eastbourne. I was interviewed and was offered the job round about June 1985 and so I sold the practice and moved down to Eastbourne.

I left practice because I'd been at it for 24 years at that stage. It was boring, not to put too fine a point on it. The other problem is that as dentists get older, the patients got older with you; you didn't attract the young patients. Well, this was my experience. I found I was dealing with the same patients over and over again. Gradually I got them to the stage where they were coming in and having nothing to do, which meant of course there was a limited income. So, there were financial implications, there's no doubt; but the financial issues I think were overshadowed by the general dissatisfaction.

Working for Dental Protection now as I do, I come across quite a number of dentists who have been at it for 15 or 20 years, sometimes longer, and they've become disenchanted with the whole thing. Some of them turn to alcohol; others become so casual about dentistry that they no longer seem to care and I think it is a mid-working life problem.[37] It certainly happened to me, and I can sympathise so much with people to whom it happens in practice. I had an ability to get out, albeit I was lucky to get out. But by and large, there's no ability for anybody to do anything else nowadays.

They don't do it deliberately. I can particularly remember one chap who I was asked to see, who had phoned up Dental Protection to say that he was aware of the fact that he was sliding into alcoholism, and I went to see him. His wife flatly refused to recognise that this was happening, which was a bit of a problem. I went to see him and he had become totally disenchanted with dentistry. His equipment was incredibly dated, and he was indeed sliding into alcoholism. But there was a thing at the time called the Sick Dentists Scheme, I think it's gone now, and he could be shunted off to Alcoholics Anonymous and the Sick Dentists Scheme, which helped him enormously and he eventually regained his interest in dentistry. So it is, I think, quite a common problem.[38]

Working for the Dental Estimates Board

So, I went to the Dental Estimates Board in Eastbourne. There were 36 dental advisors, split into orthodontics and general. I joined at the same time as two other people on the general side. I know that's going to sound silly, but it was like going back to university days. There were

---

[37] He was speaking in 2014.

[38] The Sick Dentists' Scheme started in the late 1980s but changed its name and constitution in 1991 to become the Dentists' Health Support Trust, which still supports dentists.

groups of us who would go down to the restaurant for coffee together, and it was an idyllic place to work.

The work was boring because we were being used to approve or not approve treatment, to a set of rules and we weren't really needed, we never saw patients. There was another group, the original dental officers, who would see patients, and they were actually employed by the Department, whereas we were employed by a quango, I think. But the atmosphere overcame the shortcomings.

A real problem concerned selling one's practice, assuming one had one, to move there. We were on a 12-month contract, and it was not guaranteed that you were necessarily going to have that contract confirmed at the end of the 12 months, so it was a gamble. And I'd come down from Manchester to Eastbourne; the house price differential was huge.

After a year, we all got our tickets. One chap very nearly didn't, but he was on the orthodontic side and we didn't know anything about him. Then the job improved and we started to be sent out to appeals. If we would decide not to approve treatment, the dentist could appeal the decision. And in certain cases, the appeal procedure was run by the Executive Council.[39] We would be sent out to put the Board's point of view to a panel of dentists as to whether this treatment should be approved or not, and by and large you knew you were on a loser before you went.

And then our role changed in that we became involved in probity. Probity issues had been dealt with by a separate department in the Dental Estimates Board. Clinical matters were a matter for the regional dental officers who examined the patients.[40] So, probity had been run by the Dental Practice Board, by a man called Arthur Seymour, who ran it as his own little fiefdom. The building was separate from the rest of us, and we would give our opinions and we never heard what happened to them. Then gradually that changed, so we became much more involved in probity issues, which was okay and I was in probity management for six months until I realised it was almost entirely negative work. So I gave that up.

---

[39] Executive Councils were established by the National Health Service Act, 1946 in county and county boroughs to administer the general practitioner services of doctors, dentists, pharmacists and opticians. They were abolished in 1974.
[40] Regional Dental officers carried out random inspections of work.

This was, for example, people claiming for treatment which they hadn't done. False records, occasionally false radiographs. It mostly involved finance, as you would expect. And they had disciplinary cases, and conduct hearings and we would go out and present the case. There were various penalties; they could be referred to the General Dental Council, they could be put on approval requirement where every bit of treatment, other than emergency treatment, had to be approved by the Board, which was no more than an inconvenience really but it let you keep an eye on them. I enjoyed that in a macabre sort of way.

At the time, we seemed to go through various nationalities of villains. Villains is not the right word, but when I went down to Eastbourne, the Australians were under fire. They had this wonderful term, 'bash the nash'. They would come over to the UK for a certain period and they would provide the most extreme treatment and be paid. Then the New Zealanders got in on the act, then the South Africans. This is a scandalous thing to say, but that was the case. And we used to have some happy times.

The health service record cards all had a date at the bottom of them. And it was rather jolly to go to a hearing and say, 'Are these a contemporaneous record.' 'Oh, yes, yes,' and they'd have coffee stains on them and different inks and so on. And you'd say, 'That's fine. What's the date at the bottom?' And they'd say, 'Oh, it's May 1997.' And we'd say, 'Yeah, it's interesting. You know, that's the date the record card was printed.' They'd say, 'Yes.' 'Well, how is it that treatment actually started two years before that on the record?' Now, childishly, we quite enjoyed that, so actually that revolutionised the work at the Board.

By then, our numbers were decreasing. They got rid of all the orthodontic advisors and we were gradually being whittled away. I think there was one orthodontic advisor left, a senior orthodontic advisor, and there were probably six or seven dental advisors. Then the decision was taken that the Dental Practice Board, which changed its name, could run without dentists.[41] So we were all offered early retirement/made redundant. And for the last six months, I went in 1999, I think, and there was one dental advisor there for about a year after that, and then the place ran with none.

---

[41] The Dental Practice Board succeeded from the Dental Estimates Board in 1989.

Dental protection

When I'd worked for the Dental Estimates Board, we used to travel all over the place. A particular service hearing was in York, and I had met Kevin Lewis, who was the Dental Protection chief officer. I can't remember what his title was.[42] Anyway, eventually he offered me work with Dental Protection and I've been there ever since.

I used to go into the office one day a week for about two years, which was good fun, again a very good place to work. Working with colleagues, able to speak to people and treated well. And then some other people who were part-time became full-time, and of course Stephen Hancock was there for a while. He was in the next office to me when I joined. Stephen Hancock was very helpful to me.

The Beveridge Report was the foundation of the Health Service, which was the means by which dentistry changed so dramatically. My recollection is that the Beveridge Report was made public in November 1947, saying that it's all going to be free on the 5th of July 1948, the same day they nationalised the railways.[43] And it was thought, there would be a 27 percent uptake of dental treatment in the first year. But of course, there was a hiatus between the announcement in 1947 and July 1948. Not unnaturally people thought they would hang on and get their treatment for nothing. And that was what happened, and the uptake in July 1948, I think, was in the order of 36 percent, which threw everything completely out of kilter.

The first thing the Department did was they said, 'Okay, you could only earn £X hundred a month, and anything you earn over that we're only going to give you half of.' The next thing they did was in 1949 was to chop the fees. And I've got the list of the fees. And in 1948, for instance, at the outset, you got £0.50 equivalent for an examination. In 1949, when the fees were cut, that was halved, so you then got £0.25. Dentists had been working extremely hard during that time to keep up with the demand for treatment, in effect this dammed up demand, which the Civil Service had created. And going back to the £0.50 equivalent for an examination, it isn't until one gets to 1970 that the fee becomes £0.60,

---

[42] Dental Director.
[43] The Beveridge report, 'Social Insurance and Allied Services' which provided a blueprint for social policy in post-war Britain was published in 1942. It was the 1946 National Health Service Act that provided the establishment of a health service, it came into effect on 5th July 1948.

so it took a very long time for the fees to recover. Then if we go back and look at fillings, for instance. For a large amalgam filling, in 1948 you were going to be paid £1.50, and that fee actually didn't recover until 1974. So, a splendid idea, messed up by civil servants and I suspect they didn't realise that people might stop going to the dentists.

There was a huge amount of dissatisfaction in 1949, but there was also an awful lot of money made by dentists in 1948/49. The next thing they did was introduce a thing called TARGI, by the Doctors' and Dentists' Review Board. TARGI was target gross income, and TARNI was target net income. And they would then go back, using two-year-old Inland Revenue figures, extrapolate them forwards and saying, 'Okay, your target gross income should be £60,000 and we know your expenses are, call it half – it was always more than that – so therefore the target net income should be £30,000.'

That would then be put to the so-called independent review body, and the Department of Health would veto it. The review body said what should be given, and they said, 'No, sorry, we can't afford it.' So there has always been this battle between the Civil Service and the profession. The last scale of fees, the last contract which was April 2006, has been generally accepted an unmitigated disaster, so much so that they're changing it and they're replacing it with one which appears to be an even greater disaster.[44]

They don't seem to have ever addressed the fact that there needs to be cooperation and that dentists, by and large, are reasonably intelligent and they are going to get round systems. So I don't have a lot of regard for the Civil Service, I'm sorry to have to say.

---

[44] See also: Chapter 19 for Barry Devonald's opinion and chapter 20 Barry Cockcroft who was Chief Dental Officer for England when it was introduced.

8. Gordon Fordyce

Gordon Fordyce was responsible for the introduction of vocational training for dentists. As a young dentist he treated a few facial injuries during his National Service in Austria and decided to train as an oral surgeon. Whilst he was a consultant at Mount Vernon Hospital, he became Dental Dean of the British Postgraduate Medical Federation and an elected member of the General Dental Council. I interviewed him at his home in Emsworth in 2012.

******

I think I chose dentistry because I had a good, attractive, young dentist and I think he was the one who influenced me. I thought about doing medicine but I thought no, I would do dentistry because it was a subject which I thought I could understand and that it was possible to know as much as was available about it. Whereas medicine, I thought it would have so many side-lines that I couldn't concentrate on. Dentistry was my future. The war was on and it wasn't difficult to get in, they wanted people. I was only sixteen when I started, still a young lad.

The main thing that we did, for 2,000 hours, was in the laboratory. And most of what we learned about dentistry was from a very old and very capable dental technician. He taught us more than almost anybody else.

We did a lot of dental extractions. The clinical side wasn't until we had finished our anatomy, physiology and pathology, then we had clinics that started at nine in the morning and there would be a queue of people coming to have their teeth out. It was forceps extractions, we might have had to lift a flap to get a root out, but I can't recall doing it.

I qualified in 1946 and went into general practice for a few months. We did quite a few extractions with general anaesthesia, which we administered for each other and took turns at doing the extractions.

National Service. Dentistry and facial injuries in Austria

Then my call-up papers came, and I was off to the army. I was posted to Austria. In Austria I did a clinic, in Klagenfurt and then after six months or thereabouts I was posted to the 31st British General Hospital as a number two dentist. And then when number one finished I was made the senior dental officer. And that's when I was responsible for any trauma that came in to this area of the British authority.

They were road traffic accidents and punch-ups, drunks. They were troops and their wives or girlfriends and they were in cars and they were getting their faces broken. Not a lot, but I remember one in particular, I find it difficult to forget the girl. I had a fallback arrangement that had been made by my predecessors. If in trouble, send the patient to Aldershot, where we have a hospital if they needed advanced treatments. And this girl came in with a broken face and after a day or so I thought, no, this girl had better go to where there's better treatment. And I arranged an aeroplane and a train and got her back to Aldershot and when she really woke up, they found out that she wasn't British at all, she was an Austrian girl and they didn't know what the hell to do with her. However, they got in touch with me and told me I would have to sort it out. She came back. They'd put her on splints or something.

I think I treated about four or five mandibular fractures in my eighteen months. There were quite a few loose teeth and knocked out teeth though.

Advice from the anatomy professor

So, my number came up, and I went back to St Andrews to see Professor Dow.[45] I had been interested in anatomy and David Dow was the Professor of Anatomy and he was very kind to us dental students. So, when I came out of the army, I went to see him asked him if I should do medicine. And he told me that he had been to a meeting in Edinburgh and heard that the college there, the Royal College of Surgeons in Edinburgh, was going to introduce a new examination for dentists whereby they would be awarded a Fellowship, FDS Edinburgh.[46] That would be the future and the ladder for people like me, three years training in the army, hospital experience, a little bit of Max. Fax. experience. That would be the right way and much better because I was getting on in years, and would be thinking about getting married, and going back do medicine would not be really necessary if I could pass the FDS. exam. So, I thanked Professor Dow, I had listened to him for many years and decided I would go along that path. Which I did.

---

[45] Gordon had qualified at St Andrew's University. The dental school was in Dundee.
[46] It started in 1949, a year before the FDS at the London college.

And he said that I had better do what the doctors do, and that is go back to the anatomy department and do six months as a demonstrator in the dissecting rooms. So, I set to and did this. I read my physiology at night and worked in the anatomy department in Dundee.

The fellowship had then started, this Edinburgh Fellowship in Dental Surgery. If I remember correctly, the examination was in two parts, a primary and a second part. And the primary bit was anatomy, physiology, pathology. And then once you'd passed that you could do the second part, which was clinical dentistry and oral surgery. So, I set to and worked on that and passed the primary and by that time I was ready to apply for a job. I was told that because I'd been in a hospital in the army and I had some experience, I didn't have to do a house job. I was 25 or thereabouts.

Training in oral surgery

I looked at the journals and there came a job to go to be a registrar in dental surgery at Hill End Hospital.[47] So I put an application in and was called to meet Ben Fickling, Paul Toller and Alexander McGregor who were the consultants.[48] And I was successful with this application and was taken on to start as soon as I could. And there was an Irishman, whose name I have forgotten, who was the senior registrar, full-time, and I'd be the full-time registrar and I would be able to get enough experience to sit the second part of the fellowship.

I hadn't been there many months when the Irishman, a very nice chap, had to go back home. I had done a year as a registrar and Alex McGregor said to me one day, 'Oh, Paddy's having to go home. I'll look into having you promoted to senior registrar,' which commanded a salary of £1,000 a year. The previous registrarship was £775, so this was an improvement. I was by that time married and had a son. So, I was pleased with that.

Gordon was a registrar at Hill End Hospital when the department moved to Mount Vernon Hospital in 1952, and was subsequently appointed as a consultant there. Later he became Dental Dean of the British

---

[47] Hill End Hospital was a psychiatric hospital close to St Albans in Hertfordshire and was commandeered by the Emergency Medical Services for use in WWII. It was linked to St Bartholomew's Hospital and many of the staff came from there. At the end of the war there were still many patients who needed rehabilitation. The unit provided a plastic surgery and oral surgery service to a wide geographical area north of the Thames stretching from the east coast to Oxford, so it remained in service. However, it became necessary for the hospital to be returned to its original use and the plastics and oral surgery service moved to Mount Vernon Hospital in Northwood in 1952.

[48] Alex McGregor left Hill End before the service moved to Mount Vernon to become Dean of the Birmingham dental school.

Postgraduate Medical Federation and was responsible for the birth of vocational training for dentists.

I was the postgraduate dental dean; I was chairman of the North West Thames Regional Health Authority's postgraduate medical and dental things, but my main interest was on the dental side. I had been what you would now call the postgraduate dental tutor for Mount Vernon Hospital and that area. And as chairman of the region, and particularly the dental side of it, I came across Desmond Greer Walker,[49] because he was, by that time, on the General Dental Council and looking after the postgraduate tutor side for the British Postgraduate Medical Federation, which included all the Thames regions.

He and I used to discuss the problem of the new graduates coming through and the inadequacy of the dental training that they were getting. What could we do about it and why should we do anything?

I had been, as a dental tutor, meeting a lot of dentists. Desmond said he knew, around Guildford, a good number of excellent dentists, absolutely first-class dentists; and they wished to progress, whereby they could be recognised by an examination or some sort of system and see themselves on a step on a ladder. How could that be done?

Well, I said, 'Desmond, we are very akin to the medical profession and we know that the steps there are well defined. You start off by doing your anatomy, physiology and you sit exams and you get your FRCS and you become a house officer and go up in the ladder, and it's all laid out for you. On the dental side, you can't do that. There aren't enough positions in the country to absorb a fraction of far too many.'

So, I think it was between us, we concluded that we wanted to introduce vocational training which would do something which was needed. We knew the good dentists in our areas who would want to get involved in continuing education and become tutors. There were as many dentists as there were doctors who could be good teachers; but they couldn't do it because there was nowhere they could go to teach. None or very few went into dental schools to do it. So here we had a reservoir of people, educated people, prepared to be involved in continuing training. So, there we had the start.

What we had to do was try to have a system whereby the postgraduate dean in the region would have a committee of selected people who would interview practitioners who wished to become recognised as trainers. So,

---

49 Consulting Dental Surgeon, the Middlesex Hospital.

we put out adverts, and of course there were quite a large number of chaps very happy to do it and they were appointed. We had no money, but we weren't too concerned at that stage because the trainees would be working under the NHS conditions which would provide them with a salary for what they did, albeit under the banner of the trainer. So, it was self-funding. The trainer would get something, the trainee would get something and they would come out at the end of the year with a training.

They were to be allowed one day off a week and the dental tutor in Guildford, where the pilot scheme would be situated, would produce a training programme approved by the Dean that would be funded by money from the Department of Health, through the regional health authorities, to the post graduate centres.

So, the whole thing was buttoned up, we couldn't see a flaw in it, apart from the competition from the people in the London Hospital. I forget the chap's name, who had this other idea of dividing the year into three sections of four months, and moving people around. Well, he didn't know anywhere they could go that would be any good to them.

Then the money did become an issue, we wanted a bit more money. I had a contact through one of the dental companies, big one, American-based, and I talked to him about it and I said look, I don't need a lot but it would be useful if I had something so that I could give the trainers something. So, he said that was a wonderful idea, he was happy to help, and he gave some money to get started. John Brookman was my general practice advisor, and was to be the course organiser.[50] I think that's where I needed some money for somebody like him and the thing took off.

From inception to practice, altogether I think, it took fifteen years. It's a good story. Desmond Greer Walker was pleased, delighted that we'd got this going, really. I had succeeded him as postgraduate Dean for the British Postgraduate Medical Federation. In those days the BPMF looked after London but also the UK, Scotland, Ireland and Wales.

On the medical side, they had a bi-annual conference of postgraduate medical deans. And Desmond had started it on the dental side, and the BPMF would send out an invitation to the dental deans for a meeting in London. Not only would they be asked, but the Chief Dental Officer from London and one from Scotland, one from Ireland, would be invited as well.

---

50 Peter Kaspar talks about John Brookman see chapter 9.

The dental deans liked it because they could charge up a trip to London for a day. We had them twice a year; they had no objection, and they came. They had gone through all the things I've talked about with trying to interest people in postgraduate education and they thought, having been told about our experiment, that this was fine and they said they'd go ahead.

Then we came across a snag. Newcastle didn't like it. This was a relic of the dean at Newcastle, bloody Bradlaw. He was in cahoots with Kelsey Fry and people like that,[51] they were a group. And they discussed such things, and they had never thought of this, and to have someone, not even English, a Scottish person in London suggesting that in Newcastle that they might do this! They didn't like the idea that somebody else had thought of it. No!

Desmond Greer-Walker had resigned from the General Dental Council over it. He had tried to interest them in the idea and they said no, no, none of that. We are the people recognised to provide dental education. The GDC had no say in postgraduate education of this nature, it didn't exist. The Newcastle people were upset, so I had to have long chats with one of their people who saw the light and said 'leave it to me, this is old-fashioned stuff. Bradlaw has gone.'

In Scotland I came across another snag, and I came across it in London as well, a bit. The costs of providing postgraduate medical and dental education were given by a grant from God or somebody high up to do these things and the grant was given, and the medical people understood it was for postgraduate medical education. But when someone jumped up and said, what about dentists? They said oh yes, yes, the dentists are in. But the Scottish chap wouldn't have a postgraduate dental dean appointed for Scotland because it would come out of the medical education allowance. This sort of nonsense was going on. And so the Scottish one almost said, no, I will not allow this to happen.

So, I had to point out to him the shortfall in dental education because the first two or three groups of trainees had to fill in a questionnaire of their experience during their undergraduate training. How many teeth

51 Sir William Kelsey Fry. Consulting Dental Surgeon to Guy's Hospital, Queen Victoria Hospital East Grinstead, the Eastman Dental Institute and the Royal Air Force. He was famed for his WWI military record, working with Harold Gillies on facial injuries during WWI and his role in starting dental hygienists in the Royal Air Force, the first in the UK. See: Obituary Sir William Kelsey Fry, C.B.E. M.C., D.Sc. M.D.S., F.R.C.S., F.D.S. R.C.S. British Medical Journal November 9th 1963 1206. See also chapter 3, 10, 13 & 30.

they had taken out? How many anaesthetics they had given, that sort of thing. And I had to go to the medical people and say, look, this is what we're trying to do. So they eventually said OKAY, let's do it. They tried to modify it in Scotland a little because they said, of course, the distance that people would have to come to a postgraduate centre once a week would cost us too much if they were coming from the Isle of Sky to Edinburgh. So, we sorted that out for them and they had a residential element.

The idea of being a trainer was to work in a practice with the trainee. So, once they got to know each other, they would have free access to move from one surgery to the other. The trainer could come in, help, or the trainee could say please come and have a look at this, tell me what to think. What do you think about this treatment plan? And once the medical people got the gist of this then things became much easier.

The first postgraduate medical dean for north-west Thames was keen on the idea and he persuaded the North West Thames people to put some money in. That was not serious money, one or two thousand pounds, I think. The one in the north-east Thames had gone to the London Hospital and asked them what do they think about this and they said, oh no, it's a flash in the pan. The system we suggested would be much better. So, the next I knew was north-east Thames weren't going to touch it, so I had to find a way around that.

In a way, I cheated. I rang the CDO, Chief Dental Officer, and I explained to him that I was having trouble with the Regional Medical Officer for north-east Thames. I asked him to help me. I explained all this to him in grim detail and he said leave it to me. So apparently a telephone message was sent from them to this chap who was objecting and he disappeared and he was replaced. So, it worked, but that wasn't easy, nor very pleasant. I didn't like it.

I had to persuade the Department of Health and, through them, the government, that we needed money for vocational training. And the agreement was that Kenneth Clarke, the Minister of Health, would come and discuss it. So, I had to go along and explain to him what we were doing and the value it could be, and his answer was, that the idea was supported with enthusiasm from the Chief Dental Officers to the Minister of Health and so he agreed it should go ahead with government support, as long as it was funded within resources. But that was a go-ahead, they were prepared, and I think persuasion wasn't so difficult because in those days, the dentists graduating were almost obliged to give anaesthetics and there were many people having a lot of teeth out under general anaesthetic that the hospitals didn't want. And the public were demanding treatment.

Then I tried to explain to the various financial people that this was well within resources. They weren't having to pay their trainees anything. The trainers came out of regional funds, and eventually they saw the light. But it took fourteen or fifteen years.

It became obligatory to do it if you wished to pursue NHS dentistry within the Health Service. So we had, of course, been fairly secure in that we knew all the training practices we'd recognised were providing NHS dentistry. That didn't prohibit them from doing any private work if it was there to do. A trainee could do private work if the boss, the trainer, was happy but there wasn't much of it about. It was an unusual thing to have much private practice outside the West End.

It wasn't mandatory to do vocational training until 1988. I was invited to carry on chairing the committee by the Department of Health until I retired in 1992.

I was only working part-time when I became Dean, but I wanted to continue my hospital practice because no one would recognise me as being any use if I was not a clinician. I carried on doing two or three sessions at Mount Vernon.

Gordon became an elected member of the General Dental Council. He particularly remembered the 'feasts'

Once or twice a year they would have a dinner at night, bow tie, the lot. The food and drink flowed. I can't remember, ever, at that age, ever having food like it. And the guests came from MPs, department of health, chief medical officers, dental officers all being hugely, royally entertained.

Gordon also talked about his career as an Oral and Maxillofacial Surgeon. See: The Making of British Oral and Maxillofacial Surgery. Sadler. A.

9. Peter Kaspar

Peter qualified at Guy's and joined the first pilot scheme for vocational training for dentists in 1977, before it became compulsory. I interviewed him at his home in Oxfordshire in 2013.

******

I was thwarted at becoming a vet by fairly indifferent A-level results, and dentistry seemed like a very good alternative. Medicine never really held any interest. I was always happier with animals, and in retrospect have no regrets; dentistry suited me down to the ground.

I started at Guy's in 1971 and qualified in 1975 and then did a house job there for six months. It was not really planned, more to my surprise they asked would I do it. I said yes as I had not a clue what else to do.

After that I was champing at the bit to do a bit of travelling and I was persuaded by a friend of mine to go on the hippy trail to India and Nepal, which I did at the end of 1976. I had a fantastic time and came back December 1976 looking for a new direction.

The first pilot for vocational training

I went down to the bar at Guy's, more out of habit than anything else, and met someone who said, have you thought about applying for this new scheme? It was known as the PGA scheme then, Post Graduate Assistant. It seemed like a good idea; it gave you a helping hand in the first year.

There were only eight places and I think six of them were still available, so I sort of walked into that and what really clinched it was that one position was in Chichester, which was a town I knew and liked. And also, the postgraduate bit happened in Guildford where my girlfriend was studying, so it was just tailor-made for me, it could not have been better or more convenient.

I fell on my feet because it was Keith Osterloh's practice in Chichester, which was a very good, well-established practice. He was a good dentist and very genial; he looked after me and mentored me very well. His practice was in an old Georgian building. It came with a cottage tagged on behind which the associate could live in. It couldn't have been better. I could stumble out of bed at 8.55am and be in the surgery at 9 o'clock, just perfect.

First Vocational Training scheme experience

I did four days a week in practice. The fifth day, Friday, you went up to Guildford and had a series of seminars, lectures, talks, discussions, and then the weekend was your own.

Guildford was a one hour drive up the road. I had a rusty little MG Midget, two hundred quid, and eventually acquired a small mongrel dog when a patient offered me one. I was a bit lonely so I accepted. That ultimately gave rise to an incident at the postgraduate centre. We were having a session with a psychologist and that morning my puppy had eaten a pound of Cheddar, stolen from the kitchen, and I jumped in the car with the dog. We drove up to Guildford and in the middle of his morning seminar my dog, which was sitting under my chair, puked hugely in front of the lecturer and to his eternal credit he said, 'Excellent, that's what I call feedback.'

I was paid purely as an associate by Keith Osterloh., so I got probably 50 percent of my gross for the four days. He was my boss and supervisor and I learnt from him. He was a good man; there was an understanding that I could ask questions for guidance and help.

The only major bollocks up I did was when he asked me to do an immediate denture fit for him and unbeknownst to me, he'd already taken the tooth out. He gave me the denture to fit, and in my limited world an immediate denture was you took the tooth out and fitted the denture. So I, unfortunately, took an extra tooth out and suddenly fitted a denture where there was one missing. But he was even kind about that.

Keith was very avuncular and took me under his wing and I felt safe and he even gave me his very expert dental nurse for the first six months, so she guided me through the pitfalls of life in practice.

The day in Guildford was at St Luke's Hospital. All eight of us convened there every Friday, and it was an interesting, varied selection of postgraduate work. I don't remember any hands-on stuff. It was a more theoretical, almost philosophical, year, which suited me. I have good memories.

John Brookman was the pivotal man. He supervised it, the whole day every week. I think he did a very good job. He was another genial fellow, quite relaxed and laid back about things. I remember we went to Royal

West Sussex Hospital,[52] and we looked at the prosthetics department which was doing replacement after radical surgery and that was interesting.

I remember John Brookman and the psychologist, but I don't remember who else taught us. It was 35 years ago. It was quite grown up really, there was a lot of sharing our experiences and being supportive. We were talking about our emotions in general practice and things like that.

How many sessions the psychologist did, I don't know, but they were memorable. One day he was asking what we did to relax? And everyone trotted through the usual sort of nonsense. If I remember, fast driving featured as we were young Turks in those days, and walking and sport. And we went round the eight people and said in a very psychologist sort of way 'I notice none of you have mentioned masturbation' and there's this shocked silence and John Brookman said, 'Well hang on you haven't got to me yet.'

Later we went to one of his parties so the boundaries were nicely blurred. I remember quite a bohemian party and his girlfriend ended up naked from the waist up on the floor, having body art drawn on her breasts. I was quite impressed, if this was what psychologist parties are like, I thought.

The research project was over-egging it a bit, I think; a glorified questionnaire would describe it better. But even just learning the methodology of a questionnaire is useful and I hate to say it but much as I loathe and detest the Care Quality Commission and all that it stands for, one recommendation is regular patient surveys and things like that. So, 30 years down the line, there is some glimmer of something useful there.

I thought the day release was an excellent idea. In fact, I wouldn't mind if that had been extended for my entire practising life. The coalface of general practice is quite tough and four days a week is quite enough really. It would be good to do a bit of Continuing Professional Development input on that fifth day. I really enjoy a day's course up in London, which does feed in and fire you up and increase your knowledge.

---

[52] In Chichester. It closed in 1995 and the building was converted into flats.

10. Freda Rimini

Freda joined the RAF so that she could be trained as a dental hygienist where she remained the rest of her career rising to the rank of squadron leader. She taught and examined dental hygienists. Freda was interviewed by Frank Holloway in 2013 at the British Dental Association headquarters.

******

I left school in 1951 with not really much idea of what I wanted to do. However, I found myself working as a dental nurse receptionist in a civilian practice in Hastings. I enjoyed the job apart from the Saturday morning gas sessions which were horrendous, particularly the children. I had to hold them down whilst a mask spray with chloroform was held over their noses. Then out came the teeth, off came the mask and the child was usually sick, so that was not the nice side of it. But the rest of the work I enjoyed.

Getting the sack from a dental practice

I coped with the new form work, because of course the National Health Service had just been set up. It all went swimmingly until I got the sack. I was missing from my surgery for just a bit too long, having been sent on an errand by someone else, and when I got back, the chap I was working for was in a bit of a temper. And I'm afraid I said, 'Well, if you don't like my work, then you know what you can do, sir.' And he did. That was it, I was without a job. But I had heard about dental hygienist training so I applied to the Eastman Dental Hospital, where they were training, or retraining, the WRAF[53] hygienists, who were the pioneers of dental hygiene in this country.

The RAF started dental hygiene training in the UK in 1942. They had aircrew and ground staff who needed dental treatment and there weren't enough dentists. So it was suggested that perhaps they might think of employing oral hygienists, as they called them. There had been hygienists

---

[53] Women's Royal Airforce.

in the States for years, way back, 1906, I think, was when the first ones were trained.[54]

Joining the Air Force

I knew that this course was going on. They were training civilians and retraining the WRAF hygienists. And I had a very nice letter back saying that they were ceasing training in 1954, and that the only training was to be in the RAF. So, I applied to the RAF, and in 1953 I joined as an ACW2;[55] you can't get any lower than that. I had a fantastic career in the RAF Dental Branch and retired in January of 1988 with the rank of Squadron Leader.

I did six weeks of recruit training at RAF Wilmslow in wooden huts. We had to go to the bathhouse across all the mud, so by the time you got back to the hut, you were as filthy as when you started. And then I went to RAF Halton,[56] and I did a three months dental surgery assistant course. Then I hung around in various wooden huts, doing nothing very much except cleaning.

Dental hygiene training 1953

And then I started the dental hygienist course, which in those days was nine months. I remember we started work by scraping paint from door handles in preparation for scrapping teeth, a most soul-destroying task, which went on for weeks. And after that, we progressed to carving wax teeth. I carved quite a few wax teeth, and that took up quite a lot of time. And we then worked on the phantom heads for a while, and then worked on each other, and then, after a good three months or more, we actually started on patients. A third of the course was already gone before we actually saw a patient.

We had boiling water sterilisers. The instruments were awful, I remember sickle scalers, when new, were a nice shiny colour; as soon as they were immersed in boiling water they became black. And they had very thin handles so they were most uncomfortable things to work with.

We were taught how to sharpen instruments; sometimes it worked but not always successfully. We didn't have a periodontal hoe in those days because we knew nothing about what was going on beneath the gingivae. It was entirely different from now. There was an emphasis on

---

[54] See: How dental hygienists got off to a flying start. Michael Wheeler. BDJ Teams 2018. 29-32.
[55] Aircraftwoman second class.
[56] Lawrence Oldham did basic training in the RAF at Halton. See chapter 4.

oral hygiene, but we didn't really know what we were talking about, and that went for our tutors. Wing Commander Askew, I remember saying, 'It's very important that you encourage them to clean their teeth,' because many people didn't even bother. And toothbrushes were very large and very hard and not at all the sort of thing that one uses these days.

We were training to do supra-gingival scaling and polishing and a bit of oral hygiene instruction. If the gum was flapping away from the tooth, then we removed any deposit that you could see beneath it. But the mouths that I treated then were often pretty horrendous. RAF Halton had 3,000 apprentices. Mostly, these were the boys that we worked on.

I hadn't seen a dentist until I joined the RAF. But, being a war child, I had eaten little in the way of sweets or sugary things, so I had fairly healthy dentition.

Once we qualified, we became Senior Aircraft Women, which was a big step up. But the final examination I remember very well, because my examiner was Sir William Kelsey Fry, who was instrumental in setting up hygienist training in the RAF during the War. I also met Vera Creaton, who was the very first tutor hygienist who started the British Dental Hygienists Association, so it was an interesting time.

Breaking Sir William's pencil

In the final examination, we had to treat a patient. We had a written examination where you had three different sections, and you had two questions in each section, so we had a choice. And then you had a viva, which Sir William conducted. He remembered me for years afterwards because one question, which I didn't answer, was, 'What influence does oral sepsis have upon general and systemic disease?' And Sir William asked me why I didn't answer that question. I reached across the desk, picked up his pencil, twiddled with it and said, 'Well I find it difficult to express myself where this question is concerned,' and then I broke the point off his pencil and handed it back to him. And many years later, when I was an instructor and he was still examining, he came round while I was working on a patient, and he looked at me, and I said, 'You examined me some years ago, sir.' And he replied 'I remember, you broke my pencil.'

Having qualified as Senior Aircraft Woman, I was then posted out to RAF Boscombe Down. It was an experimental flying station.

A hygienist could only practise for a local authority or a hospital; you couldn't work in private practice, and we felt that, perhaps, we were at the start of something. I joined the British Dental Hygienist Association.

At the first meeting that I went to there were only 30, and there are well over 3,000 hygienists in the country now. So, we felt, perhaps, we were a bit pioneering.

The Royal Army Dental Corps started training in 1953. And then I think the first civilian training school was Manchester, which I think was about 1957. I think it was about the same time that hygienists could work in general practice, so there were quite a few who left the military and headed in that direction.

At Boscombe Down we were very busy. We had naval personnel as well as RAF and, of course, a lot of aircrew. I did quite a lot of flying there, but that's beside the point. But again, the general dental condition was very poor. I saw a lot of cases of, which later, was called acute necrotizing ulcerative gingivitis. When I was training, it was called 'trench mouth'. Treatment was with lots of lovely chromic acid and hydrogen peroxide; it all fizzed up and turned black. It worked wonderfully, but there wasn't a lot of gingivae left afterwards.

I remember boiling water sterilisers; there were no masks or gloves then. Sometimes I had to take off my glasses and wash the blood off them. It was all hand instruments and working standing up, and there were no male hygienists. I'm still talking about the 1950s, of course. At the end of my tour at Boscombe Down, I was promoted to Sergeant, and I was sent overseas to RAF Germany.

I was stationed at Mönchengladbach Headquarters, Rheindahlen,[57] and worked part-time at the dental centre and maxillofacial unit and also part-time in a static mobile set up outside the fire stations. In the maxillofacial unit I first encountered black copper cement which cemented silver cap splints which were used to fasten upper and lower jaws together. It was terrible stuff to get off the teeth afterwards. I also used to work in the TB wards. Now that's something which doesn't happen these days.

I used to float in and out and have a look at the chaps, and have a little chat. And we had a lot of maxillofacial patients there, because we took in the Army as well, who had nasty habits of coming off motorbikes and smashing their faces up. Health and safety didn't exist then. I enjoyed my time there.

When I came back, I was posted to Uxbridge for a short while, and then I started instructor duties at RAF Halton, where I found things were

---

[57] JHQ (Joint Headquarters) of the British forces in Germany.

just as they had been when I was training. We still had boiling water sterilisers; they were still working on door handles and they were still carving wax teeth. I was only a senior NCO and not able to change things. I did that for four years.

Hygienist training in the navy

And then I was packed off to the Navy for a year to Portsmouth at HMS Nelson. They had started hygienist training, but they didn't have anyone to help as an instructor. I think the Director Royal Navy and the Director RAF had met on some occasion, and they discussed this. The Navy wanted to borrow a hygienist tutor, and the RAF thought, well who can we best do without, so they sent me!

They had one male hygienist. But they didn't want him instructing, possibly because one male and eight WRENs?[58] I really don't know. And I don't know where he trained, either. But he was not very pleased to see me, but we got over that. But again, water sterilisers, standing position, no masks, no gloves. That was 1959, and I was there for about 18 months, the first course had started.

So first I had to sort out their standing positions, because some of them were working one side of the chair, some of them were working the other, some of them were sitting on the arm of the chair and chatting to the patients nicely. I had to be very tactful and say, 'We might find it easier if you do it this way.' And they all passed, I'm very pleased to say, and I stayed on and saw the second course through, and halfway through the third course.

From there I went back to RAF Halton again. Now as a commissioned officer, it was 1970. I walked into the clinic and I looked at the door handles and I told my senior NCO[59] to get rid of them, which she did. I thought they were soul destroying; although I suppose it taught a certain amount of manual dexterity and made one's hands that bit stronger. But you could do that on the phantom head, so why door handles? I mean, we were going back to 1943, and this was 1970.

I also looked at the wax carving. I thought well, you can learn anatomy of the teeth by looking at teeth. It helped with manual dexterity, so I kept some of that. But instead of six weeks, I cut it down, and they only had to do one tooth with a root.

---

[58] Women's Royal Naval Service, WRNS, but were known as WRENS.
[59] Non-Commissioned Officer.

I stayed at RAF Halton for the rest of my career until January 1988.

Involvement of General Dental Council

The training still followed very much the original syllabus that had been set by the RAF. But of course, I took the Ministry of Health Certificate; I qualified during that period, and then I'm not sure when the General Dental Council took over.[60] But they did, and when we had final examinations, there was always someone from the General Dental Council, an external examiner.

The GDC wanted 725 hours of clinical work. And it wasn't happening, because we were spending too much time scraping door handles and carving wax teeth. So, I was right in cutting that down.

I was appointed as an external examiner for the General Dental Council, so I got out and examined in civilian schools as well. And I was on the Examining Board, so I helped to set examination questions, particularly the multiple-choice questions where you have four statements where one is obviously wrong, one is the correct answer, and the other two could be either way. I had great fun devising those.

Changes in dental health

There was so much going on and changing in dentistry during the 1970s. We had autoclaves and ultrasonic scalers came in, I think, during the 1970s.[61] Instruments were so much better, we had periodontal hoes. We went through a mania for deep scaling, root surface debridement, I think we called it.

And the whole area of dental health education has changed. I mean, it was only in the 1970s that we started talking about plaque and understanding its implications and what was going on. Tooth brushing methods had changed. I remember when I trained it was brush down on the uppers, brush up on the lowers. You said, 'As you would clean a comb,' I think that was how we were told to do it. I think from there it progressed to giving it a good scrub from side to side. Then, much later, once we understood what was going on in the gingival crevice, we taught patients to engage their toothbrush within the gingival crevice and try to

---

[60] 1958 enabled by the Dentists' Act 1957. See: How dental hygienists got off to a flying start. Michael Wheeler. BDJ Teams 2018. 29-32.

[61] Ultrasonic scalers came onto the market in the late 1950s and their use for gross supra-gingival scaling gradually increased in the 1960s and 1970s. New designs in the 1980s facilitated their use for sub-gingival work. See: Power-driven scalers: A review for practitioners. C Hughes. Dentistry today, 2008 27(1), 50-53.

get rid of dental plaque. And there was much more emphasis on diet as well.

When I was training, I think we had a half hour talk on fluoride, water fluoridation was mentioned briefly. Hardly any mention of caries. It was, 'don't eat sweets,' You certainly didn't understand what was going on, really, in the caries process. Interdental cleaning came a bit later, maybe the tail end of the 1970s, by which time, of course, we were using ultrasonic scalers as well. These days, of course, interdental cleaning is heavily emphasised; interdental brushes are quite something now.

You can see Freda in 'Drills, Dentures and Dentistry: An Oral History' a TV film shown on the BBC in 2015 now available on YouTube.

11. Stuart Robson

Stuart was a general dental practitioner whose career started with giving anaesthetics for surgery in Canada which began a lifelong specialist interest. Stuart became President of the British Dental Association and negotiated with the Department of Health over the dentists' contract. I interviewed him at his home in York in 2017.

******

I half thought about medicine and our GP at the time was a fairly grumpy sort of individual sitting writing prescriptions. The prospect of sitting writing prescriptions didn't excite me but the family dentist was a nice guy and talked to me a lot and I think that's probably how my interest in dentistry arose.

Manchester was too close to home, because we lived in Cheshire, so I applied to Edinburgh, Glasgow and Durham. Newcastle was a part of Durham University in those days, and I was interviewed there by Professor Sir Robert Bradlaw, who was the dean. I was nervous because I don't think I'd ever talked to a professor before; I'd certainly never talked to a knight. The interview was a strange affair because my A-levels were fairly moderate; they weren't brilliant, and the whole interview lasted about 20 minutes and we talked solely about cricket because I was a halfway decent cricketer in my youth. I played a bit at Old Trafford for Lancashire's second team when I was at school. We talked and talked about cricket.

At the end of the interview, in his gruff voice, he said, 'Well, I think we can offer you a place, as I understand it the university side needs a number four batsman,' and that was the end of the interview and no mention of biology, physics, chemistry or anything. He was a great one for having his 'chaps', as he called them, representing the university in different fields of activity and propagating the reputation of the dental school, spreading the gospel far and wide.

So, I pitched up at Durham University in 1959, and it was a thoroughly enjoyable time. Over the undergraduate period there were several people who were reasonably accomplished at sport, a guy called Derek Morgan who ended up being captain of England rugby and another chap Lance

Robson, no relation, was captain of the England amateur soccer team. There was quite a lot of sporting expertise in that dental school, and it was all down to Robert Bradlaw.

In those days, we got grants from the local authority so the tuition fees and all that was paid for. I got a grant towards accommodation and my parents chipped in as and when appropriate; finance was not a problem.

The training in clinical dentistry was good, and that includes everything because in those days, we did a bit of all clinical dentistry. A certain amount of orthodontics, prosthetics, quite a lot of extractions and simple oral surgery, the odd impacted eight and that sort of thing and also a certain amount of general anaesthetic training, which I enjoyed.

Oral surgery was a highly supervised regime. The Professor of Oral Surgery was Geoffrey Howe and he was an excellent teacher.[62] He allowed his students to do quite a bit, but under strict supervision. I probably did 12-15 surgicals, something like that. They were fairly carefully selected cases not outside our competency and a couple of his registrars were very good at helping. Lester Kay, who wrote a couple of books, was one of them and also good fun as well.

In restorative dentistry, we had this wretched point system. We had to acquire so many points before you qualified. It was about 300 points or something. I think you got one point for an occlusal amalgam, three points for a MOD amalgam and 20 points for a gold inlay and you had to reach these targets, and again highly supervised. The standard of supervision was good, it was done in a kindly sort of way rather than a critical way. I think most of us didn't feel embarrassed if we made a mistake. John Walton, in particular in restorative, was quite kind about how to get out of a problem if you made a cock up of it. We did anterior teeth endodontics but I can't remember having done any molar endo.

Giving anaesthetics in Canada

When I qualified in 1964, I didn't know what to do, but I vaguely thought of going to general practice. But during the year between leaving school and going to university, I had spent some time in Canada working for the British Schools Exploration Society, which took expeditions to various parts of the world. I was lucky enough to be selected to go to

---

[62] See chapter 6 for Sir Paul Bramley speaking about Geoffrey Howe.

Labrador, where I was supposed to be doing a certain amount of surveying and geology.

While I was there, I had a minor injury and ended up in a little hospital, miles from anywhere. There was this doctor who ran the hospital, and I got chatting with him and he took me round the hospital. Then after university I saw an advert in the British Dental Journal and they were looking for somebody to do a bit of dentistry in Labrador and it was this fellow who I'd previously met. I think his name was Sam McPherson.

So, I applied for this job for six months and went for an interview in London. Then I went to Canada on an RAF flight to Goose Bay in Labrador, because they didn't have passenger flights in those days. He met me off the aircraft, and we went and had a cup of tea or coffee and he asked me if I knew anything about anaesthetics? So, being young and cocky, as you are when you've just qualified, I sort of vaguely said yes. He said he didn't want a dentist, he wanted somebody who can give anaesthetics. I told him I had a bit of undergraduate training but I was far from being an expert. Anyway, I worked with him for about six months flying between Red Indian and Eskimo settlements and I spent most of my time giving anaesthetics for the Grenfell Mission which looked after the welfare of the indigenous population.

I have to confess initially it was almost a case of the anaesthetic book in one hand and the anaesthetic machine in the other until I really got the hang of it. We had a portable Boyle's anaesthetic machine and cylinders on this light aircraft. There was no intravenous anaesthetic in these sorts of places. I gave anaesthetics for virtually everything from fractured legs to childbirth, and this guy helped me enormously. Previously, he was doing his own anaesthetics and surgery, which was tricky for him. It was an interesting experience, and that was what set me on my path to having a lifetime's interest in anaesthetics.

General dental practice

When I came back, I went into general practice in Macclesfield, Cheshire, with an excellent practice owner, where I stayed for about five years. We worked five and a half days a week, including Saturday mornings in those days. We always had a half an hour in the morning nine o'clock to 9:30 and in the afternoon two o'clock to 2:30pm where it was open to all comers for people with toothaches and so-called emergencies, and then the rest of the day was taken up with appointments.

On two half days a week we had general anaesthetic sessions because in those days there was a lot of rampant dental disease. There were loads of children with bad teeth. It was pre-fluoridation, and trying to get effective local anaesthetics in some of those children was, if not impossible, certainly very difficult. So, we dealt with a lot of that with general anaesthesia. And indeed, in adults because lots of adults, in the late 1960s, had very poor oral health, which necessitated a lot of extractions and some of them were needle phobics and some were just apprehensive of dentistry.

The rest of the week was taken up with routine dentistry, conservation and prosthetics. Of course, doing quite a lot of extractions meant that there was quite a big demand for dentures.

We were working totally within the National Health Service. There might have been a very odd private arrangement where somebody wanted some special form of dentures which wouldn't be affordable under the fee scale of the NHS, but I would think 97 percent of what we were doing was under the banner of the NHS.

We had an arrangement within the practice that what we earned on the fee scale went to the practice and then the practice owner paid us 50 percent. His 50 percent went for practice overheads, laboratory expenses and of course something of a profit for the practice owner.

In the 1960s, the patients were paying very little for their treatment. I remember a big row happening, and I think it was probably about 1964 before I was involved with the British Dental Association, because the government introduced a fee for dental inspections and I think it was five shillings. We all thought it was a doom and gloom and the end of dentistry because patients wouldn't pay that sort of money; but of course, everybody survived. Then gradually, the government decided they couldn't afford NHS dentistry, so they had an escalating fee scale for patient charges and the government NHS contribution dropped back.

Hygienists weren't even thought about in those days. Ultrasonic scalers came in; I think the first one I got my hands on was about 1970 something like that. We had a good squad of dental nurses. There were very limited training courses for them. It was up to each practice to select suitable candidates and train them up

When I first started there was still the cord driven drill, but at that stage the air rotors had come in, but the cord driven drill was quite useful if we were having to remove bone in oral surgery because it's a lot slower than the air rotor type system. Air rotors were brilliant at cutting cavities in hard teeth, but we did have the facility of a slower option. So, although the cord driven drill was perhaps antiquated, for certain procedures it was useful.

In those days, I'm ashamed to say, we had boiler sterilisers about the size of a small microwave oven full of boiling water. All the instruments were carefully washed and then plunged into this boiling water for about half an hour and then dried and then put into sealed containers, ready for the next patient. Needles weren't chucked away after each injection, they went into the steriliser, I can't remember when that stopped, I think probably 1970s at a guess, but as far as I'm aware I never ever had a patient who suffered or had any consequential cross infection. It really was very primitive, but it seemed to work.[63]

Amalgam was hand mixed with a little pestle and mortar affair by the dental nurse and then loaded into a syringe gun thing, which we then put into the cavity. I'd estimate about 1968/69, they came ready mixed in little capsules which you put into a machine which vibrated and mixed them and then you just broke open the capsule and filled the gun. We never really thought about the health of the girls mixing the amalgams by hand. But none of them seemed to have any adverse effects despite the so-called poisonous effects of mercury.

Anaesthetic technique

I was always interested in this as a topic and I got myself involved with the SAAD which is the Society of the Advancement of Anaesthesia in Dentistry with a guy called Drummond-Jackson and also a Dr Bourne and Peter Holden were the names that spring to mind. I went on one or two training courses with them and I ended up as a demonstrator on some of their courses as well, which were up and down the country, predominantly in Manchester and London.

A general anaesthetic was basic nitrous oxide, oxygen and Trilene,[64] which was superseded in about 1964 by halothane, which was infinitely better than Trilene. It was easier to administer; it created more muscular

---

[63] In 1971 the Health Committee recommended to the Representative Board of the British Dental Association, 'That hypodermic needles should be used only once by members of the dental profession and disposed of in such a manner as to ensure that they were subsequently unusable'. In 1973 the Representative Board called upon the Department of Health and Social Security to provide free disposable needles to dental practitioners who work within the Health Service. See: The Prevention of Transmission of Serum Hepatitis in Dentistry. News Report. British Dental Journal July 2nd 1974. 28-30.
[64] trichloroethylene

relaxation and had a quicker recovery time. Then about that time, early or mid-1960s, intravenous anaesthetics became more commonly used, usually methohexitone or Sodium Brietal if you use the other name and Epontol[65] which was another intravenous agent, which were very good because you could get a quick induction with minimal trauma to the patient.

I say trauma to the patient because some patients, in the old days of nitrous oxide and oxygen, did not like the mask over their face because they felt restricted, they felt claustrophobic and they were just frightened of it. Whereas by giving them a shot in the antecubital fossa or the back of the hand an anaesthetic was induced in about ten seconds; the old trick of telling them to count down from ten. Very few people actually got to below four. And then you could maintain anaesthesia with nitrous oxide, halothane and oxygen.

As time went on, we became more adventurous, doing longer stuff on patients under anaesthesia. There was a lot of dental disease around and, whereas now people have an odd filling or two done, sometimes in those days some people might need a dozen fillings, a lot, and that would take quite a while. We had this technique of topping up the induction dose of methohexitone by a drip feed off a bottle into a butterfly needle on the arm. We could thereby control the dosage coming from the drip feed system and that would minimise the amount gaseous stuff. And the advantage of that was that patients had a much quicker recovery time because the methohexitone is broken down quickly and easily by the body.

And then my colleague Brian Sidebottom got much more into minor oral surgery, so that needed a different technique altogether because he needed much better access to the oral cavity. So then I, through SAAD and other organisations, learnt to do endotracheal anaesthesia, which meant that my colleague had much better access; by putting a tube down you could seal off the trachea and there was much less risk of any inhalation of blood or any other debris. We did more of that latterly. That was in the late 1960s and was the technique that I brought with me when we moved from Cheshire over to practise in York.

It was a very different technique of course because I had to use different pharmacology in the sense that you used Brietal,[66] to induce

---

[65] Propanidid.
[66] Methohexitone.

patients and then give them a shot of Scolene,[67] to paralyse the muscles so you can run a tube down without causing any gagging reflexes and then give them a shot of atropine to keep their mouth reasonably dry as well.

Having said all that, the important question is did we have any adverse effects on patients? One or two minor incidents, but I have to say frankly nothing which kept me awake at night. But the crucial thing was that we were always very keen on patient selection. Were the patients fit? If not, we wouldn't anaesthetise them in an outpatient situation because, frankly, it was too risky. But we would, providing they were fit, ambulant and followed the instructions of nothing to eat or drink for eight hours, and they had appropriate care when they got home. Common sense, really. That was followed to the letter.

We seldom referred a patient to the hospital. We did on odd occasions, but it was usually because of medical reasons rather than surgical reasons, and I was also working as a clinical assistant in the hospital in the oral surgery department. So often I'd see patients I'd referred in a hospital environment, but that was because of a medical risk. I enjoyed working as a clinical assistant because of the consultants I worked with, David Roberts and Peter Cove.

The BMA thought the intermittent Brietal technique was dangerous, but it was not particularly the BMA who brought that argument up. They raised the question, but the question really came from the Royal Society of Anaesthetists, who were apprehensive that somebody was walking on their patch. And I'm absolutely convinced that behind the scenes there was a collaboration between the College of Anaesthetists and the BMA to stop or minimise anaesthesia in dental practice and indeed in community clinics as well. Remember that it wasn't just high street practices but community clinics. I used to go round to community clinics, giving their anaesthetics as well. The row between Drummond-Jackson and the BMA, although I've forgotten the details, led eventually to two enquiries. The Spence report and the Wyllie report.[68]

---

[67] Suxamethonium.

[68] The 'Joint Working Party on Anaesthesia in General Dental Practice' chaired by Dr A Spence was followed by the 'Working Party on Training in Dental Anaesthesia' chaired by Dr W Wyllie. In 1981 there was the 'Inter-Faculty Working Party to consider the Implementation of the Wyllie Report chaired by Professor G Seward.

Working on the Poswillo report

The Spence report created a few ripples but had little impact. It was one of those reports commissioned and, as so often with Department of Health reports, it gathered dust on a shelf for the next 30 years; it happens all the time. But it stimulated a further working party, and I'm running the clock forward now to 1991, when there was an expert working party by the Department of Health or Secretary of State, on anaesthesia in dentistry sedation and resuscitation. And that was chaired by Professor David Poswillo and which I was a member of. It was a small enquiry in number, there were about five or six of us. I can't remember all their names.

Anyway, this committee sat, and we did quite a lot of analysis of anaesthesia in general practice. I think we'd probably call it outpatient general anaesthesia because it wasn't just practice; it was community clinics and even some cottage hospitals who weren't fully organised with theatres. That was a very interesting exercise. David Poswillo himself had been in practice before he went into academic dentistry, so he understood. He was a New Zealand guy, a charming man, very knowledgeable about what he was doing. And that team got on very well indeed.

One problem that we were trying to resolve was the operator/anaesthetist. A dentist giving an anaesthetic and doing the dental treatment simultaneously, which was potentially dangerous, and it led to deaths. I'm talking about over 20 to 30 years, probably five or six, perhaps ten preventable deaths, and they were all at the hands of operator and anaesthetist. And David Poswillo himself admitted to having done this himself, not killing anybody but been operator and anaesthetist when he was in practice as a young man.

So that was one issue we had to confront. We had to improve the overall safety of general anaesthesia, improve training, minimise the frequency of general anaesthesia in outpatient clinics. Perhaps encouraging the use of sedation as an alternative and improve the training of resuscitation.

We produced this report for the Secretary of State for Health William Waldegrave. We sat in his office and gave him a briefing, which he then reported to the House of Commons. That report had far more impact than the Spence report had had ten years before in the sense that it was acted on.

It was acted on in several ways. First, it made general anaesthesia for dentistry a postgraduate subject and that meant that there were obviously implications for funding more training facilities to facilitate sedation and an up-to-date regime of resuscitation training in all practices and clinics twice a year. All the practice staff, nurses, even receptionists were involved in this.

It meant that quite a lot of practices had to stop giving general anaesthesia because they couldn't fulfil the requirements laid down by the Department of Health following that report. And those practices who still carried on, and who jumped through all the hoops, had a much bigger workload. And of course, the hospital service waiting list was getting longer, and the hospitals weren't really interested in patients for routine extractions.

People like myself and Alan Hopwood, another member of the Poswillo working party, who were fairly experienced, still had to go through these hoops of training. These courses were largely done in dental schools or, in our case, a local hospital, York General Hospital. The guy who was my tutor was also a dental patient of mine and we used to go in the village pub round the corner and have a few beers and he said, 'There's not much I can teach you about this, but we've got to go through this ritual.' It was good fun, and it got me out of the practice for half a day for a few weeks. I enjoyed that, and it stopped one getting complacent and got one involved with what were the latest developments in pharmacology of anaesthetic drugs, which I think was important.

The Society for the Advancement of Anaesthesia in Dentistry

Drummond-Jackson was almost a fanatic. Perhaps fanatic is too strong a word. He was obsessive, that's probably a better phrase, of promoting intravenous anaesthesia. He wanted the easiest way, most acceptable way of making dentistry acceptable to quite a large percentage of the population who were apprehensive and frightened. And he was enthusiastic about trying to develop, in particular, intravenous anaesthesia because he thought it was better than the old-fashioned inhalation anaesthesia.

He was quite a good teacher but he was dogmatic and he wouldn't tolerate too many arguments. His way, was the best way. I can't remember the details of it but he got involved in a legal case about it and it went on for a long time.[69] He was a very pleasant chap, but he was fairly

---

[69] See Chapter 6 for Sir Paul Bramley speaking about the legal case.

entrenched in his beliefs. He got together with some other enthusiasts. This would be mid 1960s and organised various courses up and down the country.

He was the prime lecturer. Including understanding the safety aspects and patient selection. Then they had practical sessions using dummies and taught how to do injections in the arm. He was very keen on patient selection, which rubbed off on me considerably, a very helpful message. These courses must have trained hundreds if not thousands of dentists in using intravenous anaesthesia. And it was down to him predominantly, but his acolytes as well, to pursue this path with a lot of vigour.

There was an opinion that it was a quick and relatively easy way of doing massive amounts of restorative dentistry, and I'm not sure I subscribe to that view. I certainly didn't take that view from my own personal experience. We reserved that for patients who were apprehensive of, but needed, dentistry and there were many people around in those days; it's much less now. I think some dental practices may have given general anaesthesia as an easy way out for the dentist. I think there was a little element of that, but I'm not sure that it was widespread. It was a rumour that was spread and I'm not sure how valid it is.

Sedation

I used Midazolam to an extent. The other one which you hear little about these days is, was relative analgesia using oxygen nitrous oxide in a 50/50 mix, maybe half a percent of halothane which kept the patient in a twilight zone but didn't completely anaesthetise them. That was quite an effective way for children.

British Dental Association

I have been involved with the British Dental Association since the mid-1970s. Once when I went to a local British Dental Association meeting in Leeds, somebody in their infinite wisdom decided I could become secretary of the Yorkshire branch. I had little to do other than play a lot of sports, so I reluctantly agreed and then it just sort of developed. It was never an aspiration, or a planned career.

From those lowly beginnings, I was elected to the Representative Board in London and from that to the council of the Representative Board. I ended up as vice-chairman and then chairman of the council, and a whole raft of other stuff, more or less at the same time. I was also chairman of the British Dental Association's finance committee. The

British Dental Association gave me a secondment to various departments of health.

One that springs out to mind was I chaired the British Dental Association's dental man power review body, which was a big job, looking at dental manpower in the 1990s. And then I was one of the lead negotiators on the new contract for dental practitioners in the 1990s when we renegotiated the whole of the GDS contract. That was another very big job, so that's why I was up and down to London a lot. And then I ended up as President of the British Dental Association in 1999/2000 which was hard work but a good fun year.

The old practitioner contract was past its sell by date for a variety of reasons. One was about fees for anaesthesia, and there were a lot of problems with dental remuneration. Dental remuneration was based, since 1948, on payment for work done. You got a couple of pounds for this sort of filling; you got two pounds for an inspection. I can't remember all the figures, but each item of treatment was priced.

We worked out that this was wrong, and if a dental practitioner should be entitled to remuneration, it's varied through the years, of say 50,000 pounds a year, and I'm going back to the 1970s or 1980s. So, you get 50,000 pounds a year and how do you pay that? You pay that by item of treatment. So you assume that your average practitioner does so many hundred fillings, so many hundred extractions and then you break that 50,000 pounds down into components what an average dentist would do clinically. And then you'd fill in the forms each month for work done, you'd send them off to the Dental Practice Board, they would check them and rubber stamp them and send you a cheque for the amount.

That was outdated because dental treatment had changed and there weren't so many fillings being done. Dentists, in those days, got paid a gross amount of fee, out of which they had to pay the practice expenses and the staff, and so what was left was net profit.

So, we set about trying to change all this and when the thing was completed, having an item-of-service treatment was only part of it. We also gave a capitation fee based on the number of patients that you had, so much a patient, a bit like a medical practitioner, gets a capitation fee. Then we also got a lot of bolt-on goodies. We got part of the practice expenses paid directly by the government rather than through the gross fee business, and one of them was council tax on your property, paid directly by the Department of Health.

We organised a fee for postgraduate training. Before that, the dentist had to provide their own, at their own expense. Now you get an allowance direct from the government for postgraduate education. You also now get long-term sickness allowance. Before, if you were sick, you got no income because you weren't doing any work. Now you can get an income and I think I'm right in saying up to six months' income based on your previous averages. We also negotiated maternity payments for those who had babies.

None of these things were available in the previous contract. So those were all big pluses which made the financial aspect of practising life a lot easier. We also got a substantial pay increase of the gross fees and then the Secretary of State who we had a lot of dealings with, Kenneth Clark, said when we got the thing up and running that he would leave things for two years, a pilot period, to see how the new contract worked.

Our big mistake was, and I'll put my hands up to this because I was one of the lead negotiators, we did not get that in writing. Then two years later when William Waldegrave became Secretary of State for Health, he reneged on it because he claimed NHS dentistry was costing the government too much money. He cut out the capitation fee and partially reverted to the item-of-service fee and that created a lot of unrest and problems. Quite a few practices thought about going into the private route because they couldn't trust the government. I think that's a fair summary of where we were with that contract, but there was a lot of work that went into it.

Duties of President of the British Dental Association

The Chief Executive runs 64 Wimpole Street[70] and runs the staff and makes sure that the smooth running of the committees is appropriately staffed and so on. That's a simplistic view, but it perhaps gives the picture. The President is the flag waving front row outside 64 Wimpole Street. Again, that's a fairly simplistic assessment of it, but it's not too far from the truth.

When I was President, the Chief Executive was John Hunt and he and I got on exceptionally well and occasionally when there was an overlap of duties or attendance at certain things, we kept an amicable arrangement.

The presidential job meant going round the country talking to all the branches. I visited every dental school and talked to final year students

---

[70] British Dental Association headquarters

and that was more of a recruiting exercise to persuade final year students to join the British Dental Association when they graduated.

I was invited abroad. I turned down some invites because what happened in the UK was more important to me than what happened abroad. But nevertheless, I was keynote speaker at the Indian Dental Association conference in Delhi, which was an interesting experience. I went to the Canadian Dental Association, a big annual congress in Halifax, Nova Scotia. I went to two or three places in Europe, including Frankfurt, Amsterdam and had another trip to Florida. All in the cause of promoting British dentistry and in particular British dentists.

12. John Bayes

John Bayes was a general dental practitioner in Lincoln who had a special interest in dental anaesthesia, he was a disciple of Stanley Drummond-Jackson and the Society for the Advancement of Anaesthesia in Dentistry. Together with a medical GP, he successfully campaigned for the Lincoln water supply to be fluoridated. Later he became a Dental Practice Advisor and advisor to the health authority. I interviewed John at his home in Lincolnshire in 2012.

******

There was a gentleman dentist by the Stonebow in Lincoln who rented six rooms above the chemist shop. He was 82 and I went to see him to see if he was going to retire. His name was Mr Tingle, and his daughter worked with him, and she said when father decides to retire, we'll give you a ring.

Eventually, I bought the practice when Mr Tingle died. It was very run down and the equipment was antiquated. I paid his daughter £10 for the practice and then re-equipped and decorated it. I put new plumbing in. There were three rooms on the second floor, above the chemist shop and a technician on the top floor.

One wasn't allowed to advertise in those days, but I made it known that I was going to start on July 24th 1960. There were only about 15 practitioners in Lincoln of which I was the youngest, probably by about 20 years. When I opened there was a queue about 400 yards long down the High Street for people to come and sign up to become patients.

In a rural area like Lincolnshire, it was mainly extractions and dentures. I had a local consultant anaesthetist who came and gave the anaesthetics. We had three morning sessions a week taking teeth out and I should think I did about 30 full upper and lower dentures a week to replace what we'd taken out. I got very good at taking teeth out and making dentures.

I had five years in single-handed practice at that address. Then the chemist below retired and sold the property so I moved into another practice further down the High Street with Messrs Hutchinson and

Powell. They had an established practice there and Mr Powell's father had retired, so there was a place for another dentist.

Dental anaesthesia and joining the Society for the Advancement of Anaesthesia in Dentistry

My first involvement was through a very good anaesthetist I had in my early days when I was in single-handed practice. He was very interested in dental anaesthesia and we did some cases where he intubated patients in the chair. I'm talking about the early 1960s which was quite pioneering work at that time.

We did several cases for phobics where he put tubes down with the patient sitting up. I did the dentistry and he maintained them with gas, oxygen and halothane; that started my interest in anaesthesia. Then, towards the end of 1965 SAAD, the Society for the Advancement of Anaesthesia in Dentistry, came into being, mainly due to the pioneering work of Stanley Drummond-Jackson. I joined that and went to some of their inaugural meetings and became quite heavily involved.

When I joined Stephen Powell and Jeff Hutchinson, they were already doing general anaesthetics, albeit not intravenously. They were just using gas, oxygen, and halothane and I started giving them myself then. I'd had little training up to that; I'd had some as a student, which was very sketchy and I'd been on some postgraduate courses.

Early sedation with Jorgensen technique

We used a certain number of intravenous anaesthetics in the early days, given by anaesthetists who came into the practice. This was before sedation had really taken off and the benzodiazepines became fashionable. One of the early sedation techniques was the Jorgensen technique, where one gave the patient up to 100 milligrams of pentobarbitone intravenously, followed by 25 milligrams of pethidine. This worked quite well, but the patient really was sedated for a day and had to be taken home in a vehicle to sleep it off over the next 24 hours. But one could deal with a phobic that way and probably work on them for two or three hours. The shorter acting benzodiazepines then superseded that, first diazepam and then Hypnoval, midazolam.

For the Jorgensen technique, one gave the pentobarbitone until the patient's eyelids became droopy. It wasn't a very scientific technique, but it worked. Then you followed that up with the pethidine. When you spoke to the patient, there was some reaction and they could follow instructions very slowly and sketchily. But there was massive retrograde amnesia, so they couldn't remember anything that had happened. They couldn't even remember having come to the surgery, going home or anything until they woke up in bed the next morning. But it worked.

The benzodiazepines came in around the early 1970s, we started using diazepam in SAAD. In the late 1970s, the Association of Dental Anaesthetists became active, and I was involved with that as well. That was a forum where medical anaesthetists, both consultants and general practitioners who were interested, got together and swapped knowledge. We had meetings and conferences. I think that was a very good body, and we learnt an awful lot.

Intermittent Brietal

SAAD were very keen on intermittent Brietal,[71] which was a technique where you set up a line and gave incremental doses. As the patient became light, you gave them a little bit more so that the patient remained very lightly anaesthetised. I suppose I did about 20 to 30 cases of intermittent Brietal. The skill was not to get the patient so deep that they lost their swallowing reflex. One packed the throat, but obviously the packing wasn't as efficient as having a tube down. In skilled hands I think it was quite safe, but, on the other hand, I finished in a ball of sweat.

The patients thought it was wonderful, but I was very worried about the packing and the fact they might obstruct. In fact, they did obstruct; one kept relieving their obstruction. This was before we had pulse oximeters. So, you definitely had to look for the tinge of blue. Later, you relied on the pulse oximeter.

From time to time there were one or two scary moments. People stopped breathing, but I never had a patient whose heart stopped and I never had a patient who needed to have emergency backup. I think the thing to do was screen your patients very well and if any patient was slightly contra-indicated, in terms of medical conditions, then one sent them to the hospital. Before pulse oximeters I got very worried about the technique. Although a lot of other people were very keen on it, I discontinued, particularly as the benzodiazepines were really quite efficient at producing the same result. They could produce almost the same level of comfort for the patient and the operator by sedation.

I suppose the intermittent Brietal technique was used for about 20 or 25 years by some people. Brietal continued to be used as an induction

---

[71] Methohexitone.

agent for extractions and oral surgery, I continued to use it as an induction agent for extractions.

There were several consultant anaesthetists, particularly in the Association of Dental Anaesthetists, who were very helpful and very keen on the fact that we were doing dental anaesthetics. We were doing it safely; our teams were all highly trained in CPR[72] and resuscitation techniques. I had a defibrillator which I used to take around with me if I were giving anaesthetics anywhere else and a pulse oximeter. I used to take my own equipment around with me and I made sure the staff where I was working were all fully trained in CPR techniques.

I gave anaesthetics in three other practices. One I worked at on a fortnightly basis. The other two I worked at if their anaesthetists were on holiday. The Health Service anaesthetic fee was passed on to me, less a percentage for practice expenses.

SAAD, the Society for the Advancement of Anaesthesia in Dentistry, was the brainchild of Stanley Drummond-Jackson, who was a general dental practitioner. He worked mainly under the Health Service but also had private patients and became very celebrated. He started the Society really single handed; I joined in its early days. Brietal, methohexitone, was really the thing that started it off. It was such a good short-acting general anaesthetic for outpatient work; it was really quite a breakthrough. Eli Lilly produced it.

Drummond-Jackson became a household name in the profession. We all kept going off to his meetings down in London and got very fired with enthusiasm by him. He came up to Lincoln once at our behest and gave us a long lecture on the use of Brietal, and he got quite a few younger practitioners involved in Lincolnshire.

John gave an anaesthetic to Drummond-Jackson.

When he came to Lincoln he had a wobbly wisdom tooth and he rang me up and asked me if I could remove it for him. The thing that Drummond-Jackson always used to preach was giving the minimum dose. You had to make a note of the minimum dose for each patient because it varied from patient to patient. His minimum dose, I remember, was 35 milligrams and I gave him 35 milligrams of Brietal. I removed his tooth and he was awake within two minutes and said 'that was obviously marvellous, have you done it yet?' Actually, my hand was trembling a bit because I was dealing with such a prominent personality

---

[72] cardio-pulmonary resuscitation.

in the profession. He then had dinner with us and give us his talk. A wonderful character.

Seward report

The Seward report into general anaesthesia and sedation in dentistry, I think, was initiated by certain members of the anaesthetic fraternity.[73] They were not convinced that dentists should be let loose on giving patients general anaesthetics. Although I think that in some years there had been no deaths at all, somebody had kept a very close eye on the number of accidents there had been. I think for two or three years there were absolutely no deaths at all in outpatient anaesthetics. But one year there were four deaths which were prominently displayed in the press and the media and that was the catalyst which produced the Seward report.

There were people who were for dental anaesthetics and there were people who were against it. The report more or less exonerated the profession because, I think, of the four cases that had accidents, three were anaesthetics given by consultant anaesthetists and not other dentists.

The Seward report did one very good thing, which was to make it illegal to give anaesthetics in dental surgeries without two people being present the whole time, and all staff should be properly trained. For most people who were doing it properly, it didn't make any difference because that was the scenario anyway. But then later on the Poswillo report came,[74] I think, about five or six years later when again there'd been a rash of deaths in the dental chair. When I'm talking about a rash, I'm talking, I think, about four or five again in one year, although we'd had a very quiet year, probably one or zero. This initiated the Poswillo report and Professor David Poswillo was given the job of looking into it again and providing a more comprehensive report, and further guidelines.

The report said there had to be pulse oximeters present, there had to be non-invasive blood pressure monitors, etc. Also, strict training for those people who were giving anaesthetics and without that training and documentary proof they weren't allowed to provide dental anaesthetics in outpatient surgeries. This applied to medics and dentists. The only

---

[73] Royal College of Surgeons interfaculty working party. Report of the interfaculty working party formed to consider the implementation of the Wylie report. London: Royal College of Surgeons, 1981.

[74] General Anaesthesia, Sedation and Resuscitation in Dentistry: Poswillo Report: Poswillo, DE (Chairman); Standing Dental Advisory Committee. HMSO: London, 1990.

people who were an exception to this rule were consultant anaesthetists who had to have a consultant appointment in a hospital. The way it worked was you had to attend so many training sessions and you were appointed to a consultant anaesthetist who was your, if you like, guardian angel. He had to oversee what you actually did and had to make visits when you were working and see whether you were competent, and make a report on those visits. This was Richard Thornton in Lincoln.

There were three dentists in Lincoln who signed up for the course, two others and me. Richard Thornton was our, if you like, overseer and was very helpful to us. He came and watched us work and also provided us with support if we needed it. We had to have a certain level of equipment, again defibrillators, pulse oximeters, blood pressure monitors, etc. We had to provide evidence that our staff, who were working with us, were sufficiently trained in resuscitation techniques. This was very valuable. In fact, I enjoyed the course and part of the course was spending something like 20 sessions in theatre in a district general hospital where one was working under the tutelage, if you like, or support of, a consultant anaesthetist. I was actually participating in the provision of the anaesthetic for patients in hip operations or any other sort of surgical techniques apart from oral surgery. The oral surgery department and maxillofacial department in Lincoln were very helpful as well.

I retired from general dental practice at 55, but carried on giving the anaesthetics for our practice and for two other practices. Then the General Dental Council itself got involved in anaesthetics and made new rulings. This was because of the massive number of outpatient anaesthetics that were being given. I think there were two deaths in one year. It concluded that general anaesthetics should be taken out of the hands of the outpatient scenario and that any general anaesthetic should be given in hospital.

The problem with that was that the oral surgery departments in the hospital, their main job, is not to provide simple extractions for phobics and other people in a hospital scenario. It's a very expensive way of dealing with the problem and, of course, the waiting lists increased. In my practice, in Lincoln, I had had a waiting time for a general anaesthetic to take a tooth out of probably less than 24 hours.

The Poggo clinics

Colin Poggo was medically trained, but he set up these clinics when he perceived that money could be made out of setting up specialist clinics to do dental anaesthetics. I think they served a purpose, and they were very well run, but of course, the Poggo clinics ended when the provision was outlawed.[75]

The Poggo clinics were supported by Professor David Poswillo. I went to an opening of one, I think it was in Barnsley, where Professor David Poswillo came and gave a welcoming address and said how thoroughly good he thought the service they were providing was. I thought seriously about trying to provide one somewhere in Lincolnshire, but by the time we'd got our heads round this and found somewhere suitable for Colin Poggo to come, that was when the axe fell.

Getting fluoride into the water in Lincolnshire

I became interested in fluoride in the late 1950s, when I was a student because Professor Alexander McGregor who was our Dean in Birmingham, was heavily in favour. He was looking for ways in which we could reduce the tremendous incidents of dental caries, particularly in children, in Birmingham and the number of anaesthetic sessions that were being given in the West Midlands area due to the appalling state of the children's teeth.

A lot of work had been done in America on fluoridation, adjusting the level of fluoride in the water from the minuscule amount it was in some areas, to one part per million which it had been proved by the research provided a 50 percent reduction in dental caries within five years.

There had been research done, notably in Kilmarnock in Scotland, Sutton-Coldfield and in North and South Shields. These were areas of similar demography to Lincoln and had produced a 50 percent reduction in one area, the other being left as a control. There'd been a lot of research done in possible side effects and none had ever been proved at all. So, it went ahead in the West Midlands and in 1962 the council approved the introduction of a plant to provide fluoridated water supply at one part per million.

Because of Professor Alexander McGregor's enthusiasm and also that of Peter James,[76] at the Royal Dental Hospital, who was very pioneering, I got involved. As I was hoicking children's teeth out at a vast rate of

---

[75] Colin Poggo was a South African doctor came over to the UK in 1982. He started giving dental anaesthetics full-time in 1987 when he visited dental surgeries. From 1990 he set up fully equipped clinics with properly trained staff so that patients could be referred to for their treatment. He partnered with over 40 dentists during the 1990s and his company became the biggest provider of dental anaesthetics in the country.

[76] One of the fathers of Public Health Dentistry in Britain. See also chapters 22, 23.

knots in the early 1960s with three gas sessions every week, I got involved. I thought this would be a marvellous thing in Lincolnshire as I think our level of fluoride was something like 0.1 parts per million.

I found an ally in the medical profession here, Dr Roy Schofield, and the two of us started off trying to move this forward with the local council. We provided all the evidence. I got Professor James and Professor McGregor to provide me with some sort of support on how to go about persuading the local public, as well as the local councillors, to move on this. It was a hard struggle, and we went round giving talks. The British Dental Association was very helpful. They sent me a lot of slides, material and leaflets and all sorts of things, to go round and show the public. We actually went round things like Rotary clubs and particularly targeted Round Table and young people's associations and lectured to them.

Twice we went to the council with all this. But, of course, the antis were very active in the press and one particular general medical practitioner was very anti. We were up against it with that because he suggested that osteoporosis would be rife if we went ahead. It was very difficult to combat that. People who are for things tend to be apathetic, and people who are against tend to be very active. So, we had a struggle.

It went to the council and was heavily thrown out so we went on and we entered it for another council meeting about two years later and that was thrown out as well. We then went round every councillor with all the stuff at our disposal. We made appointments with them and went to their homes and interviewed them and tried to explain to them that all the fears of the people who were against it were unfounded and tried to explain to them how concerned we were, particularly about the number of children who were being brought in for, if you like, mutilation, of having teeth taken out in bucket loads.

I went to see two aldermen, one in particular, and presented him with all the evidence. I could see he really wasn't very interested. I asked him how he was going to vote. His answer was to ask me how a certain other Alderman in the city was going to vote because he always voted the opposite way to him.

Going round the councillors proved pretty valuable. I followed it up with a letter in the local press which was, again an initiative which Peter James came up with, to press the fact that a lot of dental practitioners weren't very bothered because they were making a lot of money out of what they were doing and would have longer continental holidays because of the amount of money they were making out of taking children's teeth out. That was a big factor, the jealousy factor. We can't have this going on, we'll vote for it.

The dental profession locally in Lincoln, were not very supportive. When I came to Lincoln, the average age of the practitioner was probably 20 or 30 years older than me and they weren't really very interested. In the same way, a lot of patients who were old weren't interested. I remember giving a lecture and I think that probably 90 percent of my audience were denture wearers and two went to sleep. So, there was an age factor. The other practitioners rather took the view, well if you want to do it lad you get on with it. There were one or two medical practitioners who were keen on it as well. By that time there were a couple of younger dental practitioners coming into Lincoln and they were, of course, quite keen on it.

In 1966 or 1967 it was eventually passed, that we could go ahead and in 1969 the fluoridation plant was completed and set up and in operation. As a practitioner in Lincoln at that time, I can remember seeing the benefits. By the time five years had passed from having three anaesthetic sessions a week, I was down to one. Ten years later, from doing 30 full upper and lower dentures a week, I was down to probably doing two or three.

John was the Dental Practice Adviser to the Health Authority

The dental practice adviser came into being in 1989 for each Health Authority region; there were 90 in the country. People had to apply for the position and then the candidates were interviewed by a civil servant from the Department of Health. The administrator of the Health Authority also sat in on that, plus a lay person and someone else from the profession.[77]

When I was appointed in 1989, I was semi-retired. I thought it was quite a good thing to do, an interesting thing. I was aged about 55 or 6 and I thought I'd probably got the experience to do it. I was still doing some work but then I got this unfortunate health problem, which was in 1990, but I'd already been appointed and started.

---

[77] The dental practice advisers were set up as a joint venture between the General Dental Services Committee of the British Dental Association and the Department of Health. Their aim was to 'encourage, help and advise the profession in order to bring out the good rather than root out the bad' See: Advising the DPAs. K Pilcher British Dental Journal 166 (1989) 184.

At that time, one of the things you were doing was approving treatment plans for the Dental Practice Board. So, you got things like a D reference, where the dentist asked you to come and approve or disapprove a treatment plan. This worked well, because if it was something he didn't want to do or didn't think was appropriate and the patient was cajoling him into doing the treatment, it was a way of getting a second opinion. Then there were E references which were initiated by the Board, where they thought what had been sent to them by the practitioner to be approved possibly wasn't worth approving and they wanted someone to come and actually look at the case. You could go along and say well, these teeth are waving in the breeze, they're not suitable for bridge work or you could say, I think it would be a very good course of treatment to go ahead with.

It worked very well for a time. We had a course of instruction; we went to conferences and so on, to tell us how to proceed in certain directions.

The health and safety laws were just coming in as a very important part of dental practice and we were brought up to speed with that and had to advise and inspect practices. I went round the whole county, which was in Lincolnshire considerable mileage to do, and did a morning and an afternoon each week. It was interesting work and I got to know all the practitioners very well and I found that very rewarding in most cases.

Most practitioners accepted you, particularly when they'd seen you once or twice and realised you hadn't got horns coming out of the top of your head and that you were dealing with them fairly. I was one of them, anyway.

We had to make a practice inspection on each practice on a rolling programme and every practice had to be inspected once within a two-year period. So, with 70 odd practices, that meant we had to make quite a few visits. Some of the older practitioners were very antagonistic about changing the experience of a lifetime, of burning their clinical waste in an incinerator in the backyard or things like that. I think we got through to them in the end, some of them. I found it very rewarding. In 2000, when I retired, some practitioners were ringing me and asking me for advice; having been off the clinical scene for some time, I thought it was time I gave up.

So, I retired from that in 2000, having done it for 11 years, with a year off when I wasn't well. I think it was a very good initiative and I think it was money very well worth spending.

During the 11 years, the role was considerably diluted. We lost the job of doing treatment planning. I think it was all down to money because when the Dental Practice Board went, the whole thing changed anyway.[78] So then it was reduced to one session a week.

One of the terms of reference was to sit on the LDC, Local Dental Committee, meetings and become a go-between the profession and the Health Authority. So, I thought it worked very well in that system.

You could do as much or as little as you wished. One thing I was very keen on was the training of dental nurses and so I set up a dental nurse training programme for Lincolnshire. On one occasion when they took the dental nurses National Certificate, we finished top in the country, so that was quite pleasing.

The other thing we did was to secure a training programme for young practitioners to have training in practices after they'd qualified, vocational training. I got some funding for that in Lincolnshire because all the other Health Authority areas in Trent region had been funded, but they didn't think it was appropriate in Lincolnshire. I went down to the Department for Health and lobbied for that. Eventually, after about a year's persuading, I got the funding and Professor Rothwell [79] in Sheffield was very helpful to me in that. So those were things you could do and, if you like, make things better in your own patch, if you had the time and the energy to do it.

---

[78] The Dental Practice Board was dissolved in 2008. Prior to 1989 it was the Dental Estimates Board which started in 1948.
[79] Trent regional Post-Graduate Dental Dean.

13. Bernadette Rivett

Bernadette became a dental nurse in 1940s and later secretary to Orthodontic Professor Ballard at the Eastman Dental Institute and later to the World Health Organisation Dental Health Officer. She was interviewed in her home in 2012 by Stephen Simmons.

******

I was born in Forest Gate in North East London in 1924. At the outbreak of World War II, we evacuated to Surrey and came to live in Woking. During the war I worked in the Civil Defence Service as an ambulance attendant and as a secretary to the medical officer in charge of Civil Defence Medical Services. When the war ended, I was transferred to the office of the Clerk of the Woking Urban District Council as a stenographer.

Dental Nurse in private practice

After about a year I was approached by Mr Harold Slater, senior partner of the leading dental practice in Woking (Slater and Pickering), whom I knew slightly, socially. He asked if I would like to be trained as a dental nurse/chairside assistant. They urgently needed a replacement for someone who was leaving. I accepted his offer and started my career in the dental world in 1946. It really was the best practice in Woking.

I was there for three years, 1946 to 1949. When the NHS started in 1948, it made very little difference to us because they didn't go into it. They treated nurses who were on National Health panels, that was an insurance scheme for health workers. We remained private until I left and I don't think they entered the National Health system for some time after.

Every day was different. We had a mix of patients but they were people who could afford the prices; we were the leading practice in Woking. As to the dentists themselves, I know Mr Slater had a technique of anaesthetising one tooth at a time. He made a little hole through into the bone with a little topical anaesthetic. He drilled through bone and then anaesthetised just one tooth.

We had little sterilisers in each surgery. When I look back now, I'm ashamed because I would just take the instruments off the tray, and I didn't even rinse them under the tap. I put them straight into the steriliser. There were no disposable things. Needles were used over and over again. There was hardly anything that was thrown away at all. I spent an awful lot of my time folding little pieces of gauze. I can't remember what they were actually used for.

We had X-rays. There was a little cellar, with a red light, under the stairs where we used to go down to develop them. We had general anaesthesia with gas, oxygen and Pentothal. And in those days, very often the patient would ask their general practitioner if he would come and administer the anaesthetic. Otherwise, one of the other dentists would be called in to do it.

One dentist I worked for was really quite a character. I remember going to the local hospital or nursing home to do full mouth extractions. In the middle I have known him say, 'Nurse, my hand is so tired, you do the next ones,' and I have extracted teeth. And I have also done the same with full gingivectomies under general anaesthetic. I have cut away bits of gum. I knew it was illegal, I was terrified, but I was brought up in four handed dentistry to do what my dentist told me to do, so I did it.

I decided after three years that I would like to expand my experience and get on a bit and go to work in London, perhaps as a dental chairside assistant or a secretary. I went to night school and studied my shorthand and typing again so that I could apply for jobs as a secretary, which I did. Eventually got the job as secretary to Professor Clifford Ballard, who was the head of the department of orthodontics at the Institute of Dental Surgery at the Eastman Dental Hospital.

I'd had such a happy time at the practice in Woking. It had been three years of comradeship and extraordinary experiences. When I gave my notice to Mr Pickering, Mr Slater had died by then, I burst into tears and couldn't stop crying. They had to take me upstairs to Mr and Mrs Pickering's bedroom and I sat on the bed until I recovered myself. After that, I calmed down and moved up to London to a new experience altogether.

Secretary at the Eastman Dental Hospital

My early memories of the Eastman are of an enormous enthusiasm and activity because the department had been physically bombed during the war, and had just been restored. I think it was then that the Institute of Dental Surgery of the London University was set up and the heads of the departments had just been appointed. And they were all very young, and they all had young secretaries and we all had a very exciting time because they were all trying out their new theories. The whole thing zinged; it was very exciting. In retrospect, I realise how exciting it really was, particularly in the orthodontic department because Professor Ballard's ideas were revolutionary. They were upsetting some of the really well-established ideas of the past. It was not making him terribly popular, particularly among the more senior people. He was a man of enormously strong character and he wanted everybody to understand his new theories and to go along with him, but it was proving very difficult.

In the orthodontic department there was Philip Adams who later became the senior orthodontic person in Queen's University, Belfast and was the inventor of the Adams crib, I believe.[80] The head of the conservation department was Guy Morrant. The periodontal department was George Cross. There was professor Gilbert Parfitt. I remember a Mr Lee; I think he was prosthetics . The Dean was Professor Wilkinson. Also, there were Kelsey Fry and Dr Senior.

I started in 1949, and I left in April 1955. I was Professor Ballard's secretary for all this time and because of lack of space we shared an office, so he had to put up with me typing and he had to try to concentrate with all this noise going on.

He was a very clever and kind man, very human, and was interested in all sorts of things. He was a doctor and a dentist having both qualifications. He didn't suffer fools gladly and the atmosphere sometimes could be rather tense. But everybody learnt how to deal with it because it was worth dealing with because they were all going to learn an awful lot from him.

Those who agreed with his revolutionary views were very loyal and extremely friendly, and that lasted. I was very fond of him and that lasted really all the rest of his life and we kept in touch. He spent four years asking me to go back after I had left, but one has to move on.

Secretary to World Health Organisation Dental Officer

In 1954, I thought I really had to change my job. I saw advertisements for the World Health Organisation (WHO), who were looking for

---

[80] See: The Modified Arrowhead Clasp. C.P. Adams. Transactions of the British Society for the Study of Orthodontics 1949. 50-51 (Report of a demonstration at the Liverpool Dental School).

secretaries. I applied and after a lot of tests and interviews I got a job there.

By that time I had gone up the secretarial ladder and the job at the Eastman was a good job; but at WHO I had to start again in the typing pool, and that was a rest that I enjoyed. I was one year in the typing pool. When I applied for a job outside the typing pool, the deputy director general, who was looking at the applications, sent a message back. 'This girl, should be saved because we are appointing a dental health officer and she obviously has had a lot of experience in the dental world.'

I applied for the job as secretary to the new dental health officer and got it. WHO had appointed a consultant to set up suggestions for a proposed dental health programme for the World Health Organisation; he was yet to arrive. I walked into the office and the large desk was just covered in piles of paper all over the place, and I was told to set up an office. So, I had to look through all the papers and devise a filing system and set up something to be ready for the new dental health officer when he arrived. He was Dr Carl Sebelius who was from Kansas in America and he and I really were the first people to set up this programme. The objective of the World Health Organisation is the attainment of the highest possible level of health for all peoples. So that applies to every speciality within the organisation.

Expert Committee on Water Fluoridation

We started at a very interesting time when fluoridation of water was the big question of the day. And our little programme allowed us one expert committee in one year, about $3,000 for travel and about three months of consultant help. It was very small indeed.

Dr Sebelius used most of his time getting in touch with everybody in the world that he could think of to belong to a panel of experts that could be drawn on for meetings and specialist opinion. He did this extremely well. Within a year he'd set up his contacts, and we were able to have the first dental health expert committee, which was on the fluoridation of water. This was enormously controversial at the time.

Because there were only the two of us, we worked closely. The expert committee meeting lasted a week, and the result was a report recommending the fluoridation of water supplies. That was 1957 or 1958. The report of that committee became one of the bestselling reports of

WHO meetings of all time because it was so controversial; the controversy went right down to grassroots level.[81]

The experts came from all over the world as far as we could manage it. When the World Health Organisation was set up, there were 55 members only. Now there are about 200 countries with so many countries gaining independence. We had to choose from those who were members of WHO, which was just about everybody in the world.

The person in charge in WHO would have knowledge of all the experts in their field and would choose from those. But you had to be sure that there was a proper geographical distribution, otherwise there could be conflict. There would be maybe something like eight or ten members of an expert committee and you could, for example, only have one British, one American, one French and if you were lucky, you got one from Africa and other countries that were up and coming. We made it as wide as possible and included countries that were particularly interested in a particular subject, so the American one was very useful in the fluoridation expert committee. We could ask anyone we liked, but it had to get through all the channels, up through the director of our division, the assistant director general, the deputy director general and the director general. They all had their say as things went up the chain.

There were not an awful lot of us when you think of the number of staff in WHO then, and the secretaries had power that they probably don't have nowadays. I was called up to see the deputy director general in the absence of my boss to fight for the people that my boss wanted to come to this expert committee.

We were living in Geneva and we were put into small cheap hotels until we found somewhere to live and then we were set up in little flats on our own or we shared with other secretaries. Things are different now; they recruit much more locally and with people who turn up casually, because it was quite an expensive thing to do.

I left that job in 1960 when I left the dental world and got a promotion and became secretary to a director of the division of health protection and promotion. That had various units in it such as cancer and cardiovascular diseases. But then I got another promotion to be the assistant to an assistant director general, which I did for 13 years.

---

[81] The First Report of the Expert Committee on Water Fluoridation was presented to the WHO Executive Board in December 1957.

14. Douglas Johnston

Douglas started as an apprentice technician in 1949 and described the work and training before eventually starting his own lab. He described some now obsolete techniques. He spoke with Mark McCutcheon at his home in 2012.

******

I was born in Craigmillar, Edinburgh in 1934 and we had little money. My mother broke her teeth. but you could get them repaired for nothing at the dental hospital in Chamber Street, so she asked me would I take them up. I took them and had to go back the next day to collect them. I was sitting waiting, and this guy came along and he asked if I would like to have a look at the lab. He took me downstairs, and he showed me all over the place and I thought this was fantastic. Probably, I think it was the Bunsens and the guy sitting at the bench, setting up and such like, that clicked with me. I decided I wanted to be a dental technician.

Getting an apprenticeship as a dental technician

I left school when I was 15. I went to the Labour Exchange and said I wanted to be a dental technician. The guy said no chance, but I've got a job as a blacksmith. I thought not really; I said put my name down in case something comes up. So, he kind of thought for a minute and then he said, I've got somewhere where you could have a shot and this was the Lothian Dental Laboratories at George IV Bridge. It was owned by a guy called Paddy Carr. Paddy Carr had a reputation. He was an Irishman, and he was quite volatile. He had a big lab, and he didn't have any time for anybody who didn't get a move on.

So, I went along to see him, and the interview took about 15 minutes. 'Okay, start on Monday.' He could see that was what I wanted to do, and he said to me later on that the reason I got the job was because my shoes were polished. That was 1950, just about two years after they started the National Health Service. All dental treatment was free then.

It was a big place. There must have been about 25 technicians there and six of us apprentices. I started working in the plaster room and I took messages and work to and from dentists on bikes with a basket on the front. We'd deliver messages and put the work in the basket and off we went. I call him Paddy Carr now, but then it was Mr Carr. All the technicians were called Mister, and all the dentists were called Sir in those days.

Most dental practices then had a technician, who usually worked in a small cupboard, or in the attic, or in the cellar, usually just one technician in a small room. The dentists who would have used the likes of Mr Carr's laboratory were just single-handed practices, I think. But there was such a lot of work then because dentistry was all free and the work used to come in from all over, by post. They had big plaster, setting up, polishing and filing rooms. They were big premises.

I, being an apprentice, just did pieces to help the technicians. I did what I was told and tried to learn as much as I could. I remember Mr Carr showing me how to cast impressions one day, and he had this strong Irish accent. So, he mixed up the plaster in a bowl and he said to me, 'Run under the top.' And I looked at it and he says, 'Run it under the top, boy. Run it under the top.' And I said, 'how can you run it under the top?' And then he pointed to the sink. Run it under the tap. So, it was amusing as well.

I used to work from 8:30 till one o'clock and two o'clock till six o'clock. On Saturdays from 8:30 till one o'clock. On the Saturday morning, we apprentices had to scrub the floors and everything else and if it wasn't done correctly, about quarter to one, he'd just get a bucket of water and tip it up so you were till two o'clock. It was a busy place, which suited me fine and he gave me a five-shilling rise after the first three weeks. I still only got a pound a week, mind.

Acrylic and vulcanite

The bulk of the work was acrylic work, but we still did vulcanite. We had about four or five vulcanisers, which were all polished with black boot polish and all the gauges were polished till they were shining. It was run like an army dental lab if you could imagine, spit and polish. Mr Carr was ex-army, as were most of the technicians. Most of them used to work at the army dental headquarters, which is the Gillsland Park Hotel, now.[82] They came to work for Paddy Carr when they got demobbed when the war finished.

Making vulcanite dentures was also quite a tricky procedure. They were waxed up the same as you would wax up dentures today. It was all

---

[82] He was talking in 2012.

porcelain teeth, of course, attached with little pins. There were two colours of vulcanite. You had pink for the gum and the red for the palate, which is a bit stronger, so they said.

You had to get a tile, like a big floor tile, stick it on top of a pot of boiling water and you would cut up sheets of the vulcanite into little strips and lay them on this tile so they softened. And then with a Lecron Carver and a point, the first thing you did was pack the flange, so you packed that in very carefully amongst the pins, making sure you didn't get it onto the palatal surfaces. So, you built that up and then you took the red and you packed that in the back, and you packed it into all these little holes. And you put the strips across the palate and then a couple of sheets of cellophane and your flasks. Of course, they were pretty hot as well. You gently pressed this up and if you had done it right you had the pink and red in the right place, and if not, it was quite a big job taking it off. You had to take the whole flange off and put a new flange on; but you got quite used to that. Later we thought this was daft, so we just used to pack them all in pink.

Once you'd packed your dentures in the flasks, you clamped them up just exactly the same as you do with acrylic dentures. A vulcaniser was a cylinder like a bomb, pretty thick cast metal with a heavy lid that went on the top and it was all tightened down. It had a pipe that came out of the side with a pressure gauge, two rubber tubes, one to the gas tap, one to the gas ring part of the vulcaniser. You put a little water in it and you tightened it all up, and then you lit the gas and set the gauge to what you wanted. So as the steam pressure inside went up, it changed the gauge, and as it went up to where it was supposed to go to, it cut the gas off, or reduced the gas because it was all kind of connected. Then you left it there for about an hour and that was then vulcanised. Then you let the steam out and it used to smell like bad eggs. And so then, you took it out, let it cool down and then you'd tap it out. And by this time the plaster was quite soft with the pressure and the temperature, so you dug it out and scrubbed it all up and then you filed it up and polished it. The main drawback of a vulcanite denture was the complicated technique and the danger of the vulcaniser.

Vulcanite dentures could last for years and years. They were slightly flexible but pretty strong. But the acrylics really simplified things. It was only a case of mixing it up and packing it in and squeezing it up. You had to go round every one of the teeth on a vulcanite denture because there was always a thin film of vulcanite rubber that went up the teeth; it had what you called a square edge, and you had to sandpaper and then you had a stone that was just a little smoother than the sandpaper and you'd smooth it all down with that before you polished with pumice and then whiting to put a shine on it.

Plaster impressions

In those days, they used to take mostly plaster impressions. It was quite a feat to take the plaster impressions off the model with a little hammer, gently tapping the plaster so it would crack. Well, first, we would put a separating medium on and then cast them up in plaster of stone, and then you had to tap them with this little hammer to knock off the plaster.

And thank goodness, alginates came along, which made it an awful lot easier. There was an old guy called Smithy who used to do most of the tapping off of the plaster and I don't know whether he had been a technician, but he used to just mumble all the time. I could never make out what he was talking about. After I'd been there a couple of years, eventually, I got out of him that he wanted me to give his dentures a polish, so I said fine, so he let me have them. So, he produced these two massive great dentures out of his mouth that he'd got in the dental hospital. Somebody had the theory that if they filled up all the space, then they got the maximum stability and this is what this guy had. And I said to him, 'I'll cut them down for you.' So, I cut them all down and re-contoured them and then he could speak all right.[83]

The training was working alongside a technician. He showed you what to do and then you had to pick it up pretty fast. The first tasks were all the kinds of things that the technicians didn't want to do such as polishing dentures. So, we used to have to do flasking and packing and then trim them up and polish them. We had a big bench and there must have been about 100 dentures a day going through. The technicians used to work till about nine o'clock at night and the place used to get full of steam. We soon became an expert at polishing. The technicians would do the setups and trim them, and then we got a shot to do all these things as well.

---

[83] This sounds like the 'neutral zone' technique for a lower denture which Professor Bates made me do as a student in Cardiff in the early 1970s. Fortunately for my patient an elderly common-sense GDP, Mr Lewis, used to come in to supervise us and he ground it all down so the patient could wear it.

Stainless steel technique

Then the lab started doing stainless steel work. Thinking of it now, it was quite dangerous because you had two great big containers full of die metal and counter-die metal. The die metal was slightly harder. I think it was all lead and tin.

You made these dies and counter-dies. You had this big box full of foundry sand. And you blocked out the undercuts on the model with plaster, and you rubbed it all over with French chalk. Then you put it on the base of the box, put a ring round it and packed the sand in. Then you had to lift it up and gently tap the model so it would fall out. So, you had an impression of the model in the sand. Then you put another ring, an extension ring, on top of that and you got this big ladle and you scooped up a ladle full of this molten metal and you poured that in till it was up to the top of the ring. You let it cool down, knocked the rings off, then you had your die. You put another ring on top of it and then you poured in the metal for the counter-die. And then that came apart, once you had that done you got a piece of stainless steel and a horn mallet, so you tapped as much as you could on the palate and kept trimming of the surplus metal, put it in the press, started squeezing it up carefully. If you did it too quick, it would either fold over on itself and wrinkle or it would split. So eventually you managed to trim it, and with a lot of trimming and cutting and squeezing, you eventually made yourself a metal plate.

It was quite an involved process. It was for full and partial dentures. All the retention was stainless steel gauze, which was welded on and the same with the clasps, they were welded and soldered. It was quite a complicated thing. That preceded the chrome cobalt and when that came in the stainless steel was more or less obsolete. That was in about 1955-56.

Night school training

When I started there was no college-based learning, but they started a night school in 1952 at James Gillespie's High School. And that was three nights a week, dental mechanics, theory, dental materials, and chemistry and physics. So, three nights a week we went to that. The chemistry and physics teacher were nothing to do with the dental world. The other teacher was a guy called Jimmy Laird, who worked for Dr Dyce in Inverleith Row.

We used to call him Dr Laird and Mr Dyce. He was a nice, quiet guy. Very strict or maybe supercilious, he used to take the night class and he would say, 'I'm the best technician in Edinburgh. No, I'm the best technician in Britain. No, in fact, I think I'm the best technician in the world.' And he was perfectly serious. All the apprentices from Paddy Carr's laboratory joined the night school along with the apprentices from the dental hospital.

The night school was all theory and then Paddy Carr suggested to the powers that be that he would kit out one of his rooms as a practical night school room, where we could do practical work. So, they started that one night a week, up on George IV Bridge.

We didn't really think anything about the hours. We would just finish work at six o'clock and got there by seven o'clock and then at nine o'clock you went home, went to bed, got up, back to work again. But I enjoyed it.

City and Guilds qualification

The chief technician in Paddy Carr's was Mr Sidney Wick. He said to me one day, 'My name's Mr Wick to you.' He learned his trade up in the Orkneys, and he had this theory that if you hadn't been born as a dental technician, you'd never learn it. You were specially gifted. The apprenticeship was five years, so you were qualified after five years, and then they brought in the London City & Guilds.

First you sat your intermediate London City & Guilds, which comprised two Saturdays, in the Edinburgh Dental Hospital, doing a practical exam, and then they had a big theory exam. There was no such thing as modules. Nowadays, they do modules, a bit here and a bit there and they get a certificate for each part.

I sat my final City & Guilds later after I'd done National Service in the army. The practical exam was the Dental Hospital. We had to make a chrome cobalt partial denture, cast a gold crown and do a full upper and lower setup, things like that. And I remember when I had my crown ready for casting, they were all queuing up to use the one casting machine. But there was also an old Solbrig casting machine,[84] which was like an antique, really. I had used one before, so I thought great I'll just use that and jump the queue. And Dr Dyce, he was an invigilator, spotted me using it and he said, 'My God, it is good you use one of these. I haven't used one of these for years.' And he thought this was great, somebody that could use an old machine.

---

[84] The Solbrig casting machine was made by the Amalgamated Dental company up until 1950. It was used in making jewellery as well as dentistry.

There was a Solbrig in Paddy Carr's lab. It was a pretty basic thing, really; it was just done by steam pressure. You had a kind of base and a little platform on it. And then you had a hinge, like off a guillotine. And there was another little pad up there that used to be on a little disc that you put a damp asbestos pad in. So, you put your ring on the lower platform. Once you'd heated it up, you put your gold in it and then you melted the gold. Then you put the arm down with the damp pad on it and the steam pressure forced the gold into the mould. The modern thing was centrifugal. You just melted the gold and off it went, it flew in.

After National Service, I went back to Paddy Carr. I got my old job back; it was just as if I had just been away for the weekend because I never forgot a thing.

In 1964 I was getting married and Sid Wick, he was the chief technician then, said 'come into partnership with me'. And I thought, well he's pretty well respected, so better the devil you know, so I had a shot doing that. We decided it would be an equal partnership. He knew most of the dentists and I was a backroom guy. I didn't really know the dentists.

Starting a lab in partnership

When we first started, we used to just work in their labs, we didn't have premises ourselves. We used to work at Mr Fisher's in Ferry Road; he had a small lab. Then there was a Dr Wilson and Mr Orr up just along Gilmore Place. They had a lab in their garage. Then eventually we rented premises in Balfour Street. We used that, and it was pretty busy. We built it up, and it was quite a big shop. And there was an old lady who lived in the flat around the back and when she died, we bought her flat and knocked away the wall and then made it into a big lab.

I didn't see any real future to earning any money just being employed by Paddy Carr's. I didn't really see it going anywhere. One thing that really triggered it off was when I had my City & Guilds, I went round to the Dental Hospital to get an interview for a job. And I remember Professor Watt, and I think there might have been a guy called Geddes there as well. They did the interview. So, I had to bend up clasps and various bits and pieces for the interview. Then it came down to the nitty gritty about the wages, and they were offering less than I was already getting paid. And I told them that wasn't much use to me. They tried to get some more, but they couldn't. So I didn't go there.

So, we formed this partnership, I used to work from 7.30 in the morning till nine o'clock at night and we used to just take £5 a week in the early years and we managed about a couple of weeks holiday in the summer if we were lucky. But the lab never closed.

We worked hard at it; it was a case of working hard and trying to build up some capital. And we eventually bought the premises. We just kept going. We took on a couple of apprentices like Graham and John Vallance and a lot of these other guys. But it came home that we spent a lot of money training them up and then they just left and they took customers away. They were quite right, there was no point working for me if they could do it for themselves, I would never recommend that to anybody.

One of my brothers was a plasterer and the other one was a brickie. When they saw what I was doing and I showed them how to do their books and all that, they went off and started their own companies. They had two very successful businesses, and they're both retired. Now they live away in the countryside and drive about in big Range Rovers, as all builders do.

15. Russell Hopkins

Russell described his training in Newcastle and the high standard of dress required by Sir Robert Bradlaw. He gave anaesthetics in practice in Hartlepool and worked in an out-of-date practice in Cambridge with no air rotor before working in Rhodesia where he realised he was not cut out for dental practice. I interviewed Russell at his home in Pembrokeshire in 2012.

******

I started at the Newcastle dental school in 1951. Sir Robert Bradlaw was the dean.[85] There were a significant number of students who were ex-national service people, odd people around who'd been aircrew and other things like that. So we had a mixture of youngsters and people who'd been round and seen the world. There were four or five women in the year. I think we had about 60 in the year all told.

Finance as a student

I got a County Major Scholarship which paid me 50 pounds a term, 150 a year and you had to buy your books and everything. You got an instrument grant when you became a clinical dental student and you bought your instruments. We all bought second-hand books from the previous year. Also, I used to get holiday jobs. We only had two or three weeks, or a month's holiday a year. I got jobs as a parcel porter on British Railways and as a taxi driver, I worked in a laundry and dry-cleaned eiderdowns which gave me money to have holidays and go overseas and do things like that. So, I got an education outside of dentistry in the big wide world.

Undergraduate training

Bradlaw equated dentistry with medicine. He insisted on a standard of dress; we wore undergraduate gowns to any lecture we went to. Dental students had to be on a par with anybody in terms of dress and behaviour. In fact, we wore gowns when we went to memorial services

---

[85] For more on Bradlaw see chapter 6, 8, 11, 22.

or anything else. Medical students didn't wear gowns, they thought we were quaint. But Bradlaw insisted on that.

The first year was anatomy, physiology, etc. The second was a waste of time because we did dental mechanics; we did dental pharmacology with it. I think dental mechanics bored the pants off just about anybody. We had to do set ups and cast gold inlays, and do all the stuff the mechanics did. We learnt how to make dentures from the beginning, take impressions, and then them up and all the rest of it. It was not for patients, they were all done for models and there was a senior technician training us, and I think everybody was bored to death in the second year.

Also, we had phantom heads. We started carving bits of chalk and then cut cavities in chalk teeth, and then cut cavities in extracted teeth. We used to go skiving around and nicking teeth from extractions so that we could have the right teeth to set up to do gold inlays in and things like that. So we went through this rigmarole in phantom head of doing some really rather lovely work, supervised, and all the angles had to be right, and no sharp edges and everything had to be bevelled and so on. It was good training, useful. And so, when we went into the third year, we could already do the limited clinical work that we had to do in conservation.

I was one of those chaps that was quite good with my hands and we used to get points. You got one point for a single surface filling, two points for a two-surface filling, three points for three surfaces and for gold inlays you got more points. And you got points for dentures; everything was pointed and I actually used to work faster than a lot of the people, and I was second in the table of point scorers. The guy that beat me, it was friendly fun, was Ceylonese. He got more than I and did beautiful work.

In those days we were good at extractions because we were taking a lot of teeth out. Most of us played sport on a Wednesday afternoon, but the fifth year used to do conservation work in the dental hospital on a Wednesday afternoon. But there was an extraction clinic on a Saturday morning. I don't think anyone did molar endodontics then, if my memory is correct. I think endodontics was all in anterior teeth. Endodontics in molar teeth was regarded as postgraduate.

As a student, you had to do twenty or more anaesthetics to be signed up and part of your exam would be medicine and surgery. We used to do ward rounds and teaching rounds in medicine and surgery at the Newcastle Royal Victoria Infirmary.

The fifth-year exam was essentially medicine and surgery, but it always included problems related to general anaesthesia and I was actually quite a competent dental anaesthetist. We were trained in the early days on gas; nitrous oxide, oxygen and Trilene.[86] We induced patients to a degree of cyanosis before turning rapidly to oxygen mixes to get them through the stage of cerebral excitement as quickly as we could. It was hairy stuff, but we were much better trained than most medical practitioners, who at that time were the anaesthetists for general dental practitioners.

Although we did a lot of extractions. I don't remember lifting flaps or drilling bone. I must have taken roots out and done some simple stuff. I don't think I had training in surgical procedures at that stage and don't remember undergraduates removing impacted teeth. If teeth broke, we used Cryer's and other things like that, we were adept at using elevators. I don't think I'd got onto hammer and chisels at that time; this was 1956, so it's a long time ago.

We didn't have all the sterility of everything as today. In those days, hand pieces were soaked in antiseptic solutions and then spray oiled.

Dental Practice with no air rotor

The first job I'd got was a temporary job in a practice in west Hartlepool. And because I'd just qualified, every morning I gave up to about eight to ten general anaesthetics whilst they whipped out the teeth. They picked me as the most junior person in the place because I'd just come out of Newcastle and knew more about general anaesthesia than anybody else there, and so I became the anaesthetist to the practice.

After that locum job. I got a job as an assistant dental surgeon in Cambridge. I thought Cambridge would be a great place. I enjoyed the environment and the collegiate atmosphere and the lovely pubs in Trumpington and places.

In the dental school, air rotors had come in, so we'd actually been trained in using an air rotor, and when I got to Cambridge in this practice, it was an ordinary electric dental motor, real backwards stuff. His practice was backwards, and he was backwards, even though he was relatively young. I found this physically exhausting work because the hand pieces were heavy and slow. The revs were not high, you could rapidly burn everything if you went too high, and the tooth would smoke and you knew you were going a bit fast. And the burs were not sharp, they were not tungsten carbide, they were just steel. It was bloody hard work. It

---

[86] Trichloroethylene.

was still the early days in the Health Service, and I just found this pretty awful.

Practice in Rhodesia

At the end of the year, I realised I was working like a Trojan, and paying income tax, and not saving anything because then income tax was 60, 70 percent or something. It was hopeless, and he didn't pay well, and I looked in the journal and there was a job in Southern Rhodesia. So, six weeks later I got out of the plane in Salisbury, Southern Rhodesia, having had a 24-hour flight from London Airport, stopping every two hours; in a Britannia.

I landed in Salisbury, which is about 6000 feet high, in a British woollen suit, in the rarefied atmosphere of Rhodesia. I had too much to drink almost immediately and passed out. So that was my introduction to Rhodesia. I worked in the practice in Salisbury for a year, during which they offered me a partnership.

Boring bloody job

And I woke up one day. I'd had this feeling gradually dawning on me, and I thought, I can't fill teeth for the rest of my life. I'd had two years of filling teeth and dental practice, and I just woke up and I thought, this is the most boring bloody job I've ever come across. And I couldn't cope with it.

Russell returned to England and became an SHO in oral surgery in Nottingham, went to medical school and became an oral and maxillofacial surgeon in Cardiff.

His story continues in: The Making of British Oral and Maxillofacial Surgery. Sadler. A.

16. Shelagh Farrell

Shelagh Farrell worked initially in National Health Service dental practice and later in private practice, specialising in prosthodontics. She became involved in dental politics early in her career, initially with the British Dental Association. She spoke about the issues as an elected member of the General Dental Council and at the College of Surgeons of England. I interviewed her at her home in Kent in 2023.

******

Bristol Dental School

I was at a very academic school and I don't think they thought I was very bright; they were suggesting that I did physiotherapy or radiography. But I am not very energetic and I can't do maths, so I thought I would do social science at university, which was very fashionable in the middle '60s, and become a hospital almoner.

Then my mother, who was head of the science department at Ealing Grammar School for Girls, told me about a girl who, having done arts A levels, went off to Bristol to do dentistry. And I thought dentistry would appeal to me because I love using my hands, and that's how it started. I didn't know about first BDS, and although I had done biology A level in lower sixth, and botany, zoology and geography in upper sixth, I hadn't got physics or chemistry. So, I started thinking, well, maybe I could do first BDS somewhere.

I was offered a place at the Royal Dental Hospital in London, but you had to go to Bart's then to do your first BDS, and the students said, 'They're awfully snooty at Bart's.' And when I went to Bristol, they said, 'Oh, you've got to come here, it's fabulous,' so that's what I did.

It took an awful long time, six years. There were seven medics and seven dentists doing first year. I didn't know how I would get through the physics, but they kept setting the same papers every five years, so if you looked them up, you sort of got through it.

After second BDS, there were sixty of us, and they could not cope with sixty people down at the dental hospital in the op-tech lab, so they failed half our year at the second BDS exam. I don't think the General Dental Council would ever have allowed that again. We were not allowed to resit in the September, we had to wait until Christmas, because that wouldn't have solved the problem as far as the laboratory situation was concerned. So, our year was absolutely split down the middle and I was referred six months, and it's the only time I've failed anything important in my life.

I think the teachers were all pretty good teachers actually, particularly some of the practitioners that came in. One really did admire them, because you knew they were doing it all the time and they knew what they were doing.

After qualification I did two house jobs because, probably like a lot of students, when you first qualify, you're a bit nervous about extracting teeth, and I just wanted to make sure I could do it before I went out into practice.

Professor Arthur Darling was the Dean. He used to have a surgical list each week, and when I was his SHO I used to admit the patients the day before, and then you had to be there in the morning pretty early in the operating theatre. Then it was his clinic in the afternoon, so you swallowed your lunch very quickly, and then you had to get there for half past one to send all the patients to X-ray first, before he came along. Patients were sent to X-ray before they were seen. He used to come along a bit like Sir Lancelot Spratt, his senior registrar and his registrar and his houseman, and then half a dozen students all trekking behind him. He really was a character. I remember on one occasion this lady had come in because she'd got terrible ulcers, and she opened her mouth and he pulled the lip back, and I could see her gradually rising out of the chair. He said, 'Well, I can't see any ulcers.' So, I said, 'Well, I think you've got your fingers on them, Sir' So she was not a very happy bunny. And then at the end of that long day, you had to go and have tea with him and Matron.

Oh golly, Matron was quite a character at Bristol. She had two front teeth with an enormous diastema, and they stuck out over her lower lip. But she was an excellent matron. Pity hospitals don't have people like that now. I think a lot more order would be in place.

National Health Service dental practice

I married John Farrell in 1973.[87] My father's cousin had left me some money, which was enough to put down as a deposit on a house to start as a practice, and I can remember John and I sitting in his mother's garden in Lyme Regis with a map of Bristol and a list of all the dentists on the NHS list, with some pins, to see if there was an open area, and there was, in a place called Frampton Cotterell. So, I bought a house there, put my plate up, and within six weeks I was booked up.

That's where I stayed; well, I owned, the practice for over twenty years. I was working there for seventeen and a half years.

The work was mostly very basic. Just scalings and fillings, crowns, some bridge work, dentures. John Farrell had decided to drop two sessions at the dental hospital to do some private practice, and when I first started in practice, he came out to Frampton one afternoon and he did all the denture work. That was a terrific practice builder, because he was very good at it and very quick. And in those days, the Dental Estimates Board used to give you, every year, your profile of how much and what kind of work you had done, in comparison with the rest of the country, and also with the other dentists in your area, and I realised that I was doing far more prosthetics than anybody else, either in Bristol or nationally.

The dental health wasn't bad. A lot of the people there were working for British Aerospace and so they were good. You did then also get quite a few farmers, and they were much more difficult and their oral hygiene wasn't good. And I always remember Marsh Midda, who was the periodontist at the dental hospital, saying, 'There's always two lots of people that you really can't get through to periodontally. One is the very rich, because they expect you to clean their teeth for them, and the other is the very poor, because they've got other things on their mind.'

The other thing of course was fluoride, and in those days, we were using topical fluoride on everybody that we could, and towards the end of my time at Frampton, I did notice that I was beginning to see fluorosis, so we were overdoing it. There wasn't any fluoride added to the water in Bristol, but middle-class families were giving their children fluoride tablets and we were doing topical fluoride, and I think it was just too much.

---

[87] John was a consultant in prosthodontics in Bristol.

I used to do a little bit of private work in Bristol at Litfield House in Clifton, with John, helping him, and then doing some work for myself, conservation, but not a lot. The advantage was I suppose later on one could do slightly more complicated work. Obviously, the remuneration was better, especially in prosthetics, but it was just nice to vary.

After 17 years I was getting a bit fed up and bored, and John had died in 1981, and I thought, well, if nobody's going to change my life for me, I'll change it for myself. So, I was lucky enough to get a place at the Eastman to do an MSc in conservative dentistry.

In 1990, I put my practice on the market. I've sold a practice twice in my life and each time I've hit a recession. The practice didn't sell until 1993, because I owned the building as well.

But then after I married my husband now, Chris May, and moved to Kent, after our son was born, I bought into a large private practice in Reigate, so from then on, I was doing private dentistry. We did at first treat children under the Health Service, but we stopped doing it after a time, so from then on it was all private. In Reigate you had a very different type of patient after Frampton Cotterell. It was a very wealthy population and well educated.

I bought into this partnership; there were four partners originally, in Ringley Park in Reigate, it was a purpose-built practice. It was very nice, beautifully done. One of my partners had overseen it extremely well, but of course the overheads were horrendous. We had a partners' meeting every two weeks and we had a financial meeting, a whole afternoon, once a year, and we had cost centres such as the X-ray centre and the hygienists. And every centre had to make a profit, and some of the dentists were very hot on all that sort of stuff. We had an extra nurse called a floater, because there's always perhaps one day when a nurse is ill, so you'd always got a nurse that could help you, and she used to help the hygienists too sometimes.

John Farrell's experiments

John had been appointed consultant in prosthetics at Newcastle, the first consultancy in prosthetics in the country, and then in 1966, he got the appointment in Bristol, because, I think his wife at the time wanted to move down to the south, her parents living in Devon and indeed John's parents did too. So, he came to Bristol in 1966. He lectured very widely, he was a brilliant lecturer and very amusing. He also wrote two books, one on partial dentures, which I still use.[88] I think it's excellently designed. It's now out of print, of course as is his book on full dentures, which actually was an accumulation of articles that he'd written for Dental Practice. He edited Dental Practice at one time, and he was always writing.

He did that research that showed you didn't need teeth to digest your food. I didn't know him in those days, but he got some little sort of muslin bags, and he got all sorts of different food, some he chewed and some he didn't, spat them out into these bags, with a ball bearing marker, in case he lost one, and swallowed them, and then of course examined the contents the other end, which he did down in the garden shed.

It showed what is digested with chewing and what isn't. I can only remember odd things that he said, that of all the meats, pork is the most indigestible. The fibres are much harder to digest. And of course, foods like invalid foods like sort of boring white fish and mashed potato, gets completely absorbed. He also marinated some meats and also bashed some with a mallet to see whether that aided digestion, because it broke up the fibres of the meat.[89]

At the end of the day, the answer is you don't actually need teeth to stay alive, you can manage quite well without, but life might not be so pleasurable. That's how he got his MDS.

He did want to repeat the experiment later on in life, but he'd got digestive problems by then, and his son, who was by then a doctor, said this work wouldn't be accepted because of his internal organs, so that was the end of that. I was rather pleased, I didn't want him to do it, not in a flat anyway.

Membership in General Dental Surgery[90]

When the MGDS exam came along, John Farrell was involved in postgraduate education, he was what they would now call the Postgraduate Dental Dean. He said, 'If you don't take this exam, you're a fool, and that's all I'm going to say.' So, I did it, and I was the only one

---

[88] Partial Denture Designing by John H. Farrell November 1971 and Full Dentures: A Personal View Paperback June 1976.
[89] See: The effect on digestibility of methods commonly used to increase the tenderness of lean meat. Farrell JH. British Journal of Nutrition. 1956;10(2) and: The digestibility of raw and cooked meat. Farrell JH Journal of Physiology. 1956 Sep 7;133 (3).
[90] Examination of the Royal College of Surgeons of England.

from Bristol out of seven that passed, so I was quite pleased with that. That was a fantastic exam; it's a pity it doesn't exist now.

As a result of that and meeting other practitioners who had taken the exam, we formed the British Society for General Dental Practice. It's gone now but those dentists there were good, very forward-looking practitioners, and we had marvellous meetings, really wonderful over the years.

The exam was one or two written papers, and then you had to prepare four patients. I think Edinburgh was different, but for London, you had to prepare four patients, two which you physically had to present. One of my examiners was Ian Gainsford, he came down, and Jerry Woodcliffe was the other. For the other two, they just looked at photos and the radiographs. They were looking closely at your work.

One patient I presented was a child that I didn't present physically. She'd got rampant caries, and I'd sent her into the dental hospital and they started to do pulpotomies on As and Bs, when she was three. So, can you imagine putting local anaesthetic into a child aged three? They did it under local, it was terrible, so she was untreatable. So, I got her back to the practice. Her mother said, 'I don't know what to do.' And one of my friends, who was a consultant anaesthetist at Frenchay Hospital, came out to the practice and gave her a general anaesthetic. We took out the upper As and Bs, and I put little metal crowns on the Ds and Es, and she was fine. I'd got rid of all the caries in her mouth. Then afterwards I made her a little upper denture to replace the As and Bs. That was one of my cases I thought was quite a nice case.

And you had to comment as to whether you thought the case was successful or not, so I said, 'Well no, it was a disaster to start with, but in the end, yes, it was fine.' I don't know how she carried on with her dentistry later in life, whether she was so traumatised that she couldn't cope with it anymore, I don't know.

For the other case that I didn't present physically, just the radiographs, I'd done an apicectomy and a root treatment; so, I showed that. And then the two I presented, one was an overdenture case and the other one was a six-unit bridge.

I think it was a shame, but the MGDS was discontinued I think to a certain extent – it's my personal opinion – it was ruined by the armed forces, because they used it for promotion and they gave their people time off to do their log diaries. So, these log diaries ended up like MSc projects, with references. Well, the average practitioner couldn't do that.

But when I took the exam, I just took some photographs, put them on a piece of foolscap with little corners holding the photos in, nothing elaborate, and of course the thing was typed. It was very simple. But once you start making things complicated the average practitioner just couldn't do that; and I think it ruined it really. Shame. And then of course you had vivas as well. I can't remember whether we had one or two vivas. They gave you cases to look at and you had to comment on them.

You couldn't take the exam until you'd been qualified eight years. I think it showed that you had a standard of general practice which was good. You also had to put a thing in about your practice, you had to describe it. All I can say is, those dentists that took it knew what they were doing. I would say they were – I'm not talking about myself – but they were above average practitioners. They were good.

The exam ended because people weren't taking it, and so the Faculty of General Dental Practice, which existed then, decided to stop it. Originally it was set up by the Faculty of Dental Surgery,[91] because there was no postgraduate exam except for the Fellowship in those days.

Dental Politics

When John died in '81, I really didn't want to spend time on my own, so I used to go to every dental meeting there was that was going, and there were some good ones around. For example, the Bath Clinical Society was a lovely society, we used to go to a fabulous supper there. And the BDA, and if you go to enough meetings, people stick you on committees. So, I started really with the BDA and I was section president, a long time ago, and then I eventually got elected to represent the south west on the Representative Board, and from there I stood for council.

I was the first woman ever to be elected to the council of the BDA. There was one council meeting that was quite amusing. Margaret Seward was on the council because she was editor of the British Dental Journal, but she wasn't elected onto it. She was sitting one side of me, and Peter Swiss, who was head of the Dental Defence Union, was the other side of me. Margaret was giving her report, and I was sitting with my chin on my hands, and suddenly I dropped off, and of course my elbows fell off the table. So, there was a bit of a kerfuffle, and Margaret turned round and said to the chairman, 'I think Mrs Farrell's had a fit.' And Peter Swiss said, 'Margaret, would you keep your voice down, Mrs Farrell's trying to sleep.'

---

[91] of the Royal College of Surgeons of England.

Then at the end of the meeting in the afternoon – Geoff Garnett was chairing it – I put my hand up to make a point, and somebody said, 'That was number two on the agenda this morning, Shelagh.' So, Geoff Garnett said, 'Will, somebody put Shelagh back in the teapot'. Oh dear! So, that was the BDA.

Margaret Seward was a great lady. She was very encouraging of people to do things, she really was. She invited me to talk at a symposium, 'Women in Dentistry' at the Royal Society of Medicine. That was in 1987, and then in 1989 she asked me to speak at the FDI [World Dental Federation]in Amsterdam, and that was called 'Room at the Top, a Profile of Women in Dentistry'. So, she was very encouraging.

General Dental Council

My first husband, John Farrell, was a member of the General Dental Council from about 1975 until he died in 1981, so I was invited, of course, once a year to these wonderful dinners, which I think have been mentioned by other people that you've interviewed. They were fantastic dinners. Until I had seen that other people had talked about them, I thought it was something that one probably shouldn't mention, because no doubt they were paid for by all the punters out there.

But I do remember the first dinner I went to. The port was 1947, which was the year I was born, that was quite astonishing, so it wouldn't have been cheap. And there was a gentleman there, the maître'd with white gloves on, clapping his hands so everybody moved together. I always remember Freddie Hopper, who was quite a character, he was Dean of the dental school in Leeds. His wife was Swedish, or Norwegian, quite a large lady, I don't mean fat, she was tall. I can remember her storming in one day with her flat shoes and a long dress, because 'hor' Freddie, as she called him, wouldn't get her a taxi. They were such characters, these people. And Arthur Darling's wife coming in with rather a low dress on and she looked as though she'd put the talcum powder tin down her front. Perhaps ladies did that sort of thing in those days. They were marvellous dinners.

Eventually I was elected to the GDC in 1986 to 1991, then I was not re-elected, and then in 1994 one place became available because Margaret Seward was elected as the president. So there was a by-election and I got in again, and Derek Seel,[92] who had been a previous dean of the Faculty of Dental Surgery, got very upset about this, because in those days it was

---

[92] Consultant orthodontist in South Wales.

not first past the post, it was transferrable votes, so I got the votes as I went along.

So, I got in and he didn't, and he wrote a sour grapes letter to the British Dental Journal saying how he didn't think this was on, that I'd got in and he hadn't. Silly chap really. But he was all right really, He just said 'We haven't got an orthodontist on the GDC.' And I said, 'Well, there's enough of you, why don't you just put a name forward and they'll get on?' which of course they did after that. So anyway, I got on, and then there was another election, because I was only there for the last two years of Margaret's five-year term, and I got in again, so I served for twelve years on the GDC. It was an interesting time.

In 1996 to 1998, we had a constitution review group. Every university had a representative, usually the dean. London of course originally had five dental schools, but they only had two people representing them. And in 1975, there were only seven dentists elected for England, two for Scotland, one for Northern Ireland and one for Wales, but after our review in 1998, there were fourteen elected dentists from England, and of course most of them were practitioners. So, I think the council in those days was an excellent council because every university was represented, every royal college was represented, and by '98 you had a dental auxiliary representative. In the early days, you had two people from General Medical Council, but we had no reciprocal membership on the GMC from us, so we got rid of them. It didn't seem like they should be there really. And there were more lay people. You had so much knowledge there.

The GDC in the '70s did not look at bad work. The Conduct Committee met twice a year, usually for only one day, possibly two, and the only things they were looking at was sex cases and deaths, anaesthetic deaths, things like that. Nobody came up for doing bad work, so that changed, and that was for the good.

I sat on the Conduct Committee between 1987 and 1991, and 1999 and 2001, quite a long time. I also sat on the Health Committee between 1994 and 2001 and I chaired it at one time for a bit. Jenny Pinder helped really move that forward, because when people had health problems, they used to come up before the Conduct Committee and it wasn't always right. The Health Committee cannot take you off the register. It can only suspend you or put conditions on your registration, so it's a much more humanitarian type committee, I think, than the Conduct Committee.

It was usually alcohol or drugs, those are the ones that you have to say, 'Well okay, you can't work on your own, you've got to have somebody else on the premises,' and you've got to say, 'See your psychiatrist regularly,' and they give their reports. Or if you've got a drug problem, they'll no doubt say you've got to go for tests regularly. What I didn't like about the Health Committee was the way they used to say what you should do. In other words, 'You have to go to the AA' or 'You have to go to the Doctors' and Dentists' group.' Now, I don't think it's for a committee like that to say. It's for their specialist people to tell them what to do. But it was a good committee, it was rather more humanitarian and it did deal with some sad cases of dentists that had just gone off the rails a bit.

An interesting thing about those committees, in Frank Lawton's day, was that we used to break at lunchtime and have a jolly good lunch. You'd have a drink before lunch but I never had an alcoholic drink before lunch if we were working in the afternoon. And then you'd have wine with your lunch. Well, when Ros Hepplewhite came along, she stopped all that. Sir Frank Lawton would have a gin and then he'd have a couple of glasses of wine. He was in his seventies, he didn't seem to wear glasses, he sat there all afternoon, he was sharp as a button.

At that time discussion came about specialist lists, and I was very much in favour of that, because Harley Street is an address, it's not a qualification. There were people claiming to be specialists when they hadn't had any appropriate training, and I just didn't think that was right for the public. So, I was very much in favour of specialist lists, and indeed wrote an article in the British Dental Journal about that.[93] During the debate, I can remember somebody saying, 'Well, endodontics is not a specialism.' So, I got up and said, 'Well, I don't know how you can say that because it is in the States, and there's a practice only a hundred yards down this very street that all they do is take endodontic referrals,' and that was Stock and Nehammer so they did make endodontics a specialism.

The other debate I remember is about the use of the title Doctor, which Margaret wanted introduced, and I didn't want it. I didn't see why we should be called Doctor. And the vote went against it to start with, and Ronnie Laird from Birmingham rang me up and he said, 'Shelagh, will you change your mind? We're going to have a vote again.' I said, 'No,

---

[93] Specialisation in dentistry. Farrell S. British Dental Journal. Jan 1989. 166 P 34.

I won't change my mind. I don't believe in it.' There was a new lay member of the council who came from Inverness, I think, and she clearly didn't believe in it, and she, in her inaugural speech, and she was a lawyer, said, 'I can see this coming up in the local papers, what a load of wallies'. I just thought that was hilarious. Anyway, but it did go through.

Margaret Seward, was a great role model and she did a lot of reforms in the GDC, which were good. And of course, it was during her time that they stopped allowing general anaesthetics in practice.

I sat on two cases on the Conduct Committee where children had died in practice, probably intermittent methohexitone, although one child I do remember, they did get her round, but then she went to hospital and was given something else that killed her.

Those cases were distressing, to see the parents there, and the children were just having a few teeth out, perhaps for orthodontic reasons, and they'd died. So, we had a vote in the council which stopped all that, and of course once you've voted, it has to stop immediately. You can't have an interim period, because somebody could die in the interim period and the legal people would say, 'Well, what are you doing? You've voted against this. You've got to stop it now.' And I can remember phoning Reigate and saying to Stuart Averil, one of my partners, who did a lot of oral surgery, 'Stuart, you've got a list this afternoon, are you doing any GAs?' But fortunately, he was only doing sedations.

Of course, there were the Poggo clinics that existed for general anaesthetics;[94] I believe Margaret had terrible letters from people saying that she'd wrecked their careers, and I think it was a difficult time for her, but she was quite right to do it. There was a lot of opposition I think from the profession, when I say a lot, I don't know what sort of percentage, but I do remember Ros Hepplewhite, who was the registrar, saying that Margaret had had awful hate mail at that time. I suppose for practices that were doing it, it was very difficult. There are kids that need general anaesthetics, and you haven't got the dental equipment in operating theatres, so how do you treat them? What do you do? I mean, if you're just doing extractions, that's one thing, but like that child I was telling you about earlier for whom I got an anaesthetist to come to my practice.

---

[94] See also chapter 12 concerning Poggo clinics.

That would not have been allowed now. So, how do you do the conservative dentistry on them? I don't know.[95]

Faculty of Dental Surgery of Royal College of Surgeons.

The Faculty of Dental Surgery in London set up an advisory board in general dental practice in 1982, and I was on that board. And from that board, I was elected onto the FDS board, which I sat on for four years, from 1987 to 1991. And then of course we decided to break away from the FDS and form the Faculty of General Dental Practice because most of the things that were being discussed on the FDS board were not relevant to general practice at all, it was hospital stuff. And so that's how I got involved in that.

So, I was on the FGDP board from 1992. All in all, I can remember sitting on committees nonstop at the Royal College of Surgeons for thirty-five years, which is extraordinary, because normally there's a time limit on these things. But these committees kept changing their names, so you went from one thing to the other. I was on the FGDP board from 1992, from when it started, until 2017, and that was good.

We saw some changes there. The MGDS was got rid of eventually, which I thought was a great shame. And, of course, the FGDP decided to leave the Royal College of Surgeons to form a College of Dentistry, which is not perhaps taking off as quickly as it might, which I think is a pity. But I guess people would join it if it had the royal status in front of it, which they will get, I'm quite sure, in due course.

And of course, we had a joint exam, the MJDF, membership of the joint dental faculties, the Faculty of Dental Surgery and the Faculty of General Dental Practice. And of course, once we broke away, the FDS said, 'Right, that's it,' so that exam for us disappeared, and I think that's a shame, because I don't really understand what's going on now, to be honest. It seems a muddle.

---

[95] A detailed report of Margaret Seward's time as President of the General Dental Council including the dinners, the lunch drinks, the title of Doctor, general anaesthesia decision and the following hate mail can be found in her book: Open Wide- Memoir of the Dental Dame.

17. Roy Walton

Roy started as an apprentice dental technician in the mid-1950s. He talked about his training and work, starting his own independent laboratory and the innovation in vacuum fired ceramics with John McLean. He was interviewed by Brian Williams in 2019.

******

When I was at school, my ambition was to be involved in metalwork and engineering. The headmaster decided that it would be a good idea if he pointed me toward being an apprentice to a dentist, as a technician.

I went to a private practice in Epsom. The practice is still there at 12 Church Street. It was a purpose-made practice with a purpose-made laboratory on the back of it, with their own caretakers who lived in. The dentists were Belgium refugees and they had obviously been impacted by the second world war. There were two technicians working in the back-room laboratory.

That was 1955. The Health Service was beginning to be accepted by dentists. I don't think every dentist was obliged to take on Health Service patients but we had a throughput of quite expensive dental work and a mixture of National Health work as well.

Technician training

My initial training involved getting models ready and cutting them up, all done with a guillotine. You'd have like a cutting board and a big knife with a curved blade on it that was hooked under a restraining point on the cutting board. Then you'd have the models that had been cast up and you used the knife to trim them round, which was really exciting. But in my second year, we had an innovation called an easy-cut, which was a grindstone with a water feed on it that washed away the sediment. That was a big labour-saving improvement. The apprenticeship was five years.

My National Service should have been during my apprenticeship but there was an option to delay it. Delay was better because it didn't interrupt your studies and learning. However, my birthday is the 4th of

June, and in 1960, when I finished my apprenticeship National Service had been abolished on June 1st, so I missed it by four days.[96]

During that time, I was given day release to go to Borough Polytechnic, I enjoyed that. I used to cycle there from Epsom. There wasn't a great deal of money in being an apprentice dental technician and I used to get the train fare paid for me. They allowed me to keep the train fare, which I thought was reasonable. My salary in 1955 was ten shillings and sixpence a week.

The City and Guilds was the standard examination at the end of your studies. I passed that and then embarked on an advanced certificate for crown and bridge work, which was an interest of mine. I interrupted that study because I got married in 1960 and we had a lovely daughter, Kim. We just couldn't make ends meet, so I abandoned dentistry and moved into a factory. The basic pay wasn't significantly different, but they paid overtime. The factory was Siebe Gorman's, who specialised in underwater diving equipment.

Eventually I realised that I didn't really like working in the factory all that much. It's funny, dentistry has a call, it has a pull. I had the idea to carry on my studies and get the advanced certificate in crown and bridge work, I had been at the factory for four years.

Crown and bridge ceramics

I decided the best way to advance my studies would be to seek a job in crown and bridge work. I went to see Chip Morgan. He was an advanced ceramist down in Malden. Chip Morgan was one of the establishments in the laboratory world and he wanted me to start at even lower wages than I was before. I had another interview, which scared the pants off me because it was with JP Brown in Surbiton, a very old establishment. They questioned me on my abilities and on why I wanted to take the job, etc., which went well. And then they presented me with a quotation that was required by a client and asked me how I would quote for it. I'd been out of dentistry for four years and having to quote for anything was something I'd never been involved with but I looked at it anyway. I said what I thought and they engaged me.

I went into their ceramic department; they expected you would make four porcelain jacket crowns in one day, where you adapt a platinum foil and then build up an alumina core. Four crowns a day is, by today's

---

[96] Conscription into the armed services started in 1939 and ended gradually between 1957 and 1960.

standards, very low. But the equipment was very old. We used to have a Ross furnace, which was a tiny little furnace which you looked into it to see what the porcelain was doing by opening the door and looking through it and shining a light on it to see what the glaze was like. And their equipment was even older than the Ross furnaces. It used to have a big control on the front of the furnace with little brass couplings which you moved around and gradually got it hotter and hotter. They had a tiny aperture and you could only fire one or two crowns at a time.

They encouraged me to carry on studying, taking City and Guilds final advanced examination, I passed that in 1971. The work that I was doing at the Borough Polytechnic was not the way it was being done at JP Browns. The thinking was totally different. One thing that I could see was totally wrong was the way they made the gold frameworks to support porcelain. You were taught implicitly that the gold supported the porcelain. The porcelain only had a compression strength, it didn't have any other attributes, apart from its aesthetics, of course. And so the frameworks that they were making just didn't fit the bill. So I decided it would be quite a good idea if I did my own thing and started my own lab.

John McLean and vacuum fired ceramics

Some of that was brought about when I first met John McLean. Then I worked for a really nice practice, a dentist, Mr Samson, who was in upper High Street, Epsom. And they encouraged participation in study groups.

One of the study group venues was the old workshop that I'd worked in back in my apprenticeship days. John McLean came down with his technician and introduced us to vacuum investing. The investments would be normally mixed as carefully as you could, but there were always pits in the casting. Dick Gale, John McLean's technician, came down and introduced us to this vacuum system that they'd got, which involved water pressure. It would have been a Venturi, I suppose, that pulled the air out of the mix. That was the first time I met John McLean and his technician Dick Gale.

Starting as an independent

I decided that I'd start something on my own. I was still working as a technician at JP Brown's and we had a little tiny cupboard which we used to use as a cloak cupboard in our house, and I converted this little cupboard with a little bench with a little motor and one thing and another. Initially, I was collecting repairs from two or three practices. I would do that on my bicycle. I would cycle to work and then do a round tour, twice a day, because I'd do the work at night. I dropped the work off and then pick it up again on the bike.

Several people were using my services, and then word spread. I was still doing the repairs, but I was really looking for crown and bridge work. In the first days after I'd given my notice to JP Brown's, I was at home with only a few jobs, not enough to fill the day, and looking at the phone, willing it to ring.

Dentists, like anybody else, talk to each other and so the service became popular, and it wasn't long before I was actually renting premises and started taking on staff. One was Dick Gale, who was Mr McLean's technician. He worked for me, and for a long time as well. I didn't take on any more than two or three staff because the premises could not accommodate any more than that. After about four years, it was apparent that I needed something quite a lot bigger. And this lovely old Victorian house came up for sale and eventually the purchase was made and I converted the bottom half of the premises to a laboratory and lived above the shop.

It grew from there and eventually I had twenty-three staff. That was the most I ever had. But that wasn't all technicians. It included people like drivers and cleaners.

Financial problems and repricing

At one point, I can remember the laboratory was actually dibbing into its reserves to stay in business. We weren't making any money at all. My daughter had qualified as an accountant and our son-in-law is also an accountant and I asked them for advice. And Kim, my daughter, gave me a really nice analogy. She said, 'Dad, there are two ways you can go broke, you can carry on doing what you're doing now or you can just get a deckchair and sit at the end of the garden.'

So, we sat down and made a price list that reflected the work that we were doing. I was obviously in contact with quite a lot of the other laboratory owners. We concluded to get the quality of work that we wanted and we were comfortable with, a technician was only capable of doing one crown in one hour. So, we expected an eight-hour working technician to be producing eight crowns a day. And we priced it accordingly. There were technicians that actually applied to work for us who said that they could do double that. But that wasn't what we were about.

There was never an intention to exclude NHS work, it was just we had to charge a price that reflected what we were doing. And yes, it did impact on the amount of work that came to us via the NHS. It didn't hurt the business; it actually flourished. We had very good relationships with a lot of the dentists that we worked for within the health system, although they were not personal friends. And obviously they were probably put out by it, which wasn't comfortable. But it doesn't do anybody any good to go broke.

McLean was right in his pursuit of new materials. One of his predominant themes in his lectures was that if you do your work properly, it might take longer and therefore be more expensive, but it outweighs doing bad dentistry that doesn't last very long. If it lasts longer, it's better for the patient, and it's cheaper in the end. And I think that was one of the predominant thoughts that came into my psyche.

When the old air fired porcelains that we had been using were replaced by vacuum fired porcelains, the aesthetics just flew. The exclusion of air was not wholly responsible, but certainly made a lot of difference. And taking the air out also improved the strength; you got a much stronger crown. Materials improvements have just gone through the roof.

Courses and seminars

We always introduced the technicians to courses, whether they were in this country or whether they were abroad. The business would fund that as a part of ongoing progress; and it paid off. We were always looking to be as proactive as we possibly could. In fact, one thing that helped the business was that, at the conclusion of the courses, we could come back to the profession, and say, these are now available through this firm and it seems to be an extremely good way of proceeding with this or that treatment.

To that end, we used to hold small seminars in the laboratory. We also invited dentists, that were interested, to come and see what was going on and we did demonstrations so that the profession had as close an insight as possible.

Later I can remember going to one of the dental exhibitions and seeing composites. And I thought we might as well close the doors now. But fortunately, they weren't so advanced that we needed to be that concerned about it.

18. Barry Devonald

From a bad start in general practice Barry was inspired at an IV practice in London and started a purpose-built practice in Lincoln. He described the issues relating to building a new practice, his involvement in SAAD and local dental politics. I interviewed him at his home in Coleby, Lincolnshire in 2022.

******

The dentist who treated me when I was a child seemed a very nice chap and he seemed to enjoy the work he was doing. I had a bent towards doing something involved with medicine and I thought that dentistry would probably be a good thing to do.

At the time I applied, you didn't have to go through UCAS[97], so you could apply to as many dental schools as you wanted. My education was in South London so I applied to Guy's, King's, and the Royal Dental. I thought Guys might be interested in me because I was sort of associated with it, having been the head choir boy at Southwark Cathedral, right next to it, but they wouldn't even interview me.

I went for an interview at the Royal Dental, in Leicester Square. The building wasn't very nice at all, it was pokey. And I went down to King's, they had just got a brand-new dental school, opened that year. That seemed nice, and they offered me a place. In those days, they would take you just on minimum university entrance exams. I went in with very low A levels, just three passes, but they were just enough and I was very grateful for that.

Dental School.

Dental School was good; we had this lovely new building which was next door to the main hospital. There were about 40 of us in each year. The dental and medical students, physios and nurses all mixed a lot. It

---

[97] The Universities Central Council on Admissions, UCCA, replaced individual applications to universities from 1961, the London medical and dental schools did not join the scheme until 1967. In 1993 it merged with the Polytechnics Central Admissions System to form the University and Colleges Admissions Service, UCAS.

was like a campus down in Camberwell and we had a really good time. We had to work reasonably hard, compared to what one sees university students generally doing; we had all the clinical work as well as all the theory. The staff that taught us were generally nice people, especially the dental technicians who taught the technical work; they were always up for a bit of fun.

I felt it was very much like doing an apprenticeship. You did something, you were watched, and you carried on doing it until you got it right. It wasn't like some university courses where you get half a dozen lectures a week and don't do much else. Our weeks were very full.

The second BDS was done at King's College on the Strand. The idea was that we were supposed to get a feeling of being at a university. Well, in fact, we didn't get that because as soon as you said you were in the medical faculty, the other faculties didn't really want to know you. And the hospital, especially if you did any sport, and I played rugby, would come and say we want you to play for the hospital, so start getting involved with the hospital right now. Which we did.

Once you got your second BDS, you went to do clinical in Camberwell. They threw you into seeing patients, not necessarily just dental patients; you had to do two weeks on casualty. And you did anything that came in. You were generally taught by the students who had done one week longer than you. They were not experts in anything, but they'd done it for a week, so they were near experts. We would be plastering up broken legs, taking foreign bodies out of eyes and facial suturing. The sisters used to prefer the dental students doing facial suturing because they felt they did it with a bit more care. But then we would also do things in the emergency room where people were coming in with heart attacks and other emergencies. So, you got a very broad experience of medicine. And that was great fun. You lived in for the whole fortnight and you were supposed to be there 24 hours a day, for the fortnight.

The relationships we had with everybody else in the hospital were good. We were a relatively small medical and dental school so we knew a lot of the medical consultants as well as the dental consultants. And of course, we had our general surgery, dermatology, anaesthetics and things like that. So we got to know them as well as our own dental specialists. It was a good time.

Practical experience.

They were keen that you should do as much as you could. And the first thing I ever had to do on a patient in conservative dentistry was a class 4 gold inlay on an upper central, a direct wax up in the mouth, which I would never want to do ever again. It was a very challenging thing to do for the first thing I did on a patient.

The fillings were all measured by points according to the number of surfaces. So, you would get three points for an MOD. You then had different points for gold or porcelain work. And off the top of my head, I think we had to get something like 1500 points before you could take finals. But nobody ever had any problem getting that number up because we were in an area where there was a lot of conservative dentistry that needed to be done. We got very good teaching in prosthetics and a good grounding in orthodontics. We had child patients; we didn't do any of them under sedation or anything like that. Later on, in my career a lot of my children were done under inhalational sedation.

Resident house job.

I qualified in 1971 and did a resident job for the maxillofacial department, I didn't do any conservative dentistry or anything like that for six months, I was just doing surgery. I worked for three consultants, John Sowray, who was head of department, Malcolm Harris, and Geoffrey Forman. I got a good deal of experience of different techniques, because they all had different ways of doing things, which was very valuable.

From my memory, we only had one senior registrar and two registrars. When we were on call, you were the first on call and they were at home and they would have to come in if needed. One senior registrar, who lived down near East Grinstead, did say that it was a long way for him to come in so could I possibly manage to do everything without calling him?

It was hard work. There were two of us covering the department as residents, and you went on call at 12 o'clock on Wednesday lunchtime and you came off at 12 o'clock on the following Wednesday. You did all the operating theatre sessions, inpatients requiring any dental care, all the consultant outpatient clinics, and then A & E in the rest of time, in the evenings and weekends. At weekends we ran a couple of clinics just for dental pain. But we were encouraged not to take teeth out because otherwise they felt that we would be overwhelmed with the number of people coming in to have extractions. It wasn't satisfactory, but we did take teeth out. In an A & E session you could see 20 to 30 patients on a

Saturday afternoon, and then the same sort of number on a Sunday morning. Meanwhile we were trying to cover the rest of stuff that came into A & E.

I was lucky that there were a couple of medical students who were qualified dentists doing medicine. So they were able to deal with a lot of patients that didn't need operative stuff done to them, without calling me. Although they did call me for some interesting things.

I got called one time to see a chap with his foreskin stuck in his zip. I said that it was not my area of expertise but he thought that the best way to get the zipper off was to cut it off with an air turbine. 'You've got a mobile air turbine, haven't you?'

I was introduced to the patient and he obviously thought I was an expert in foreskins in flies' zips. So I went away and got the mobile air turbine kit, which was a nice little trolley with a Borden box on it; the turbines at that time were fairly new. It was powered by a compressed air cylinder so I wheeled in an air cylinder, at which point the patient was looking at the cylinder and I think he thought I was going to use an arc welding torch on him or something like that. But we connected it all up, I reassured him and we actually just cut it off quite comfortably for him. He was quite amazed, as was I.

Because of that, word got around that the resident dentists could do things with air turbines. And another time a postman came in; he'd 'fallen' and got his penis and one of his testicles through the handle of a pair of scissors. The tissues had all swelled up, and they tried to get a ring cutter under to cut through the handle, but they couldn't. So yet again the air turbine came into use. A child with a finger stuck in a kaleidoscope was another air turbine job. And all these things could generally be done without any local anaesthetic. An interesting little side-line.

Although it was hard work, in those days there was a lot more camaraderie around. At about 11.30 at night sandwiches were always brought into A & E for everybody who was there. And you'd sit down with other people, if you'd got time, and chat. And because you were living on site, you got to know all the other housemen, who you'd been training with in any case. It was a great experience. I was there for six months.

Dental Practice.

I then went to practice in Chertsey, where they were advertising for two associates. I went with a colleague, who I qualified with, and had been doing the non-resident house job at King's. The principal, who was

133

a chap in his early 70s, had a position for three associates. The practice was in a lovely house in the middle of Chertsey which had previously been his home. It turned out not to be a good move. We didn't get any advice about choosing dental practices at dental school; we didn't get out to see practices as they do nowadays.

When we told him that we had been trained to do conservative dentistry seated, we were offered kitchen chairs so we bought our own dental stools. The dental chairs were the old type 'sit-up & beg' chairs not suited to supine dentistry.

We weren't going to get any further in our careers there; the principal was outdated in his techniques. Once when he had gone away on holiday, we were getting low on burrs; the diamonds were getting completely worn out. So, we went to try and get some out of the stock cupboard, but he'd locked it, so we got into it to get some fresh burrs. And while we were in there, we realised that he'd been using burrs and when he felt they weren't good enough for him, he put them back in the packets for us to use.

I worked there for a year and I was genuinely dissatisfied with general practice. I was not sure if I could carry on working like this for the rest of my career. So I thought about going back and doing oral surgery. I went back to see Professor John Sowray, and he told me to go for it. But he also said that I would probably have to think about doing medicine. I wasn't keen on going back and doing a medical degree. We'd just got married, and Beth, my wife, was doing her medical house jobs.

By chance, I went on a SAAD[98] anaesthesia and sedation course, just before I left Chertsey and we were tutored in groups. The two dentists who were tutoring our group were Ian Brett and John Harrison, both Australians who ran a practice out in Walthamstow. They had been featured on a Panorama programme, which was running dentistry down; 'digging for gold' and 'Australian trenches' were brought into the programme. They got quite rubbished on it.

They told us that we would know who they were because of the TV programme, and all the furore that has happened around it. They said we would get to know them over the weekend and invited us to go and see their practice so we could judge for ourselves what they were doing. So, just before I left Chertsey, it was the day after we'd given a leaving party

---

[98] Society for the Advancement of Anaesthesia in Dentistry.

to all staff, to which the principal refused to come, I went with Stuart, my friend who I qualified with, up to Walthamstow.

The practice really blew my mind. It was situated in an old cinema and it had been completely refurbished in a very modern way that I had never seen in a dental practice. I thought it was fantastic. Both Ian and John had got a lot of American influence and good design into the practice. Today, if you went into the practice, you'd think it was a very modern practice, but then it was fantastic. They were doing a lot of the dentistry under anaesthesia and sedation and we watched them do the work. The slickness of it all and the good treatment they were doing impressed me enormously.

They asked me about my career and where I was going and I told them I was just about to start a series of locums, because I didn't really know what I was going to do. And they said they'd got a position coming up in October, and would I think about coming to work with them? Of course, I thought that was fantastic. So, I did locums for a while and then I went to Walthamstow. In Chertsey I wasn't advancing in any way of learning new skills, and I just thought this is going to be a dead-end life in general practice. But then Walthamstow was a completely different experience. I was the only UK trained graduate and the rest were all antipodean.

I worked there for two and a half years, and I spent a lot of social time with them, which was great. A lot of Australians would come over immediately after qualifying and earn a good income working in the NHS, and they enjoyed life to the full. Ian and John offered me a partnership there. But I could see that I would have always been a junior partner, they'd been together for probably nearly 10 years by then.

Setting up a new practice.

At dental school, we were in small firms of six guys and girls. We went through all our training in that group, that firm, and we always used to say that wouldn't it be great if we all set up in one big general practice together, because we all got on well. But things move on and young people qualify, move away to where they came from and get married. It ended up with three of us thinking that we would create our own dental practice. We wanted a new practice; we didn't want to buy anybody's goodwill. And we wanted to build a purpose-built dental practice.

But Ed, one of the guys, then got married, and there was no way his wife was going to leave Yorkshire. Rick Newton was a very close friend of mine, and still is, and he came from Lincolnshire. And because we wanted to squat in a purpose-built practice, we needed to be sure we could have a good number of patients. Lincolnshire at that point was one of the most under-dentisted places in the country, so we decided Lincoln would be a good place to set the practice up.

Rick's grandfather and two uncles ran a building company in Lincoln, called Barker and Sons. The Barkers had some land where they were going to put some four-bedroom houses, it was in an area where there was a tremendous amount of new housing and so we bought some of that land for a practice.

While I was still working in London, Rick came and joined me for the last six months to get some experience in doing IV sedation and anaesthesia. The anaesthesia we were using was intermittent methohexitone and sedation was Valium, diazepam.

So, we were now two of us who wanted to do this project. And we had really high ideals of what we wanted. So we went round to try and raise some money for this because we didn't have enough money ourselves, obviously. We approached loads of financial institutions, London banks and other finance houses. And the general comment from them was, well, what you're trying to do is too big to start off with. Perhaps what you ought to do is get a surgery on the first floor in a high street. You know, nearly always above a dry cleaner, near a bus stop and start off and build up. And that was the very environment we didn't want to work in.

We were getting a bit despondent about raising the money, and we came to see some banks in Lincoln and got the same response from them; they really didn't want to know. Then it was suggested that we should try the Nat West Bank, right in the middle of Lincoln, the Smith's Bank it was called, to see if they would help.

So, I contacted the bank manager, as one could do in those days. I got through to him and outlined what we wanted to do, and he agreed to see me. We were working all week in London so the manager suggested we meet him in the Mint Street club, the gentleman's club in Lincoln at eight o'clock on a Saturday night.

We were in the corner of the snooker room giving our presentation, and Rick and I got it to be reasonably slick by then. The bank manager showed no emotion whatsoever. So, under my breath, I said to Rick, 'we've failed here, let's just be polite, and we'll go and have a beer'. But then the bank manager said that although he couldn't sanction the amount we wanted to borrow, because it was more than his limit, he would make phone calls on Monday morning and give us a call. And he did phone us, and said that we could have the money. So then we could go to the architects and the builders and start doing some detailed work.

We started off, and we were going big. We wanted four operatories, fully equipped for sedation and anaesthesia, a hygienist surgery and a separate examination room, because we felt that it was good for patients to be examined in a room where there wasn't a lot of dental equipment. It was to have a dental chair and dental light, and that was all that was needed to make it comfortable. And we had a fifth surgery that we didn't equip. We had a central sterilizing room, which was unusual in those days, and that was fully equipped with ultrasonic cleaners and autoclaves. There were three recovery rooms, staff facilities, staff changing room, and a lounge area, which everybody said was much too big because it was 40 feet by 40 feet with the reception on one side. We always called it the lounge area because waiting room implies, you're going to wait, whereas lounge sounded a little bit softer to us. And so, the practice was built.

The building was raised three-foot six above ground level so that all the services could run underneath it. We had compressed air, hot and cold waters, waste, and piped anaesthetic gases run into the five operatory surgeries. We didn't need it all in the hygienist's surgery or the examination room.

We built two flats on top, because we were putting everything we'd got into this. We thought we'll put some flats on top where we could live. When we were more established and everything was going okay, then perhaps we could move out of the flats.

We came up from London and opened the door in January 1975; we had put in a receptionist the month before. In those days you couldn't advertise, but the builders had put a sign up outside saying Barker and Sons Builder, Washingborough. And in about three-inch-high letters along the bottom it said 'Proposed New Dental Surgery'. Well, it didn't take long before we got a call from the GDC because they'd gone to the builders to find out who had commissioned them to do the building, and they came to us and said that we were advertising and had to get it down straightaway. So we had to take the 'Proposed New Dental Surgery' off it and we wondered whether it was a local dentist who might have complained about it. We opened on the fifth of January, 1975.

Rick's dad was a great raconteur. He liked going to the pubs and he would chat to people. So, he was going around pubs and saying, 'They're building down Doddington Road, I was told it's going to be a dental surgery.'

The receptionist, who came in December, had never done dental reception work at all. But all she had to do was book people in for examinations, starting on January 5. We were concerned that we wouldn't have enough patients initially. So, we had backup that we could go back and work in the practice in Walthamstow one or two days a week should we need to. But we were never near having to do that.

We were each seeing over 100 new patients a week. And we carried on doing that for some years. It was fairly hectic, especially as being in a very under-dentisted area. There were people who hadn't been to dentists for ages and they needed a lot of work doing. It was a great help that we were used to doing sedation because you could get people in and find out why they hadn't got dentistry done. Perhaps they couldn't get into a dentist or because of phobias and a dislike for dental treatment. We thought sedation was a justifiable way of providing treatment for people who had phobias, or just a dislike of having dentistry done.

The best advertisement we could ever have was to have a happy patient, because they told all their friends. We were just inundated with people coming in. Patients often needed very many fillings and perhaps also extractions to be done and that was going to take weeks of coming back backwards and forwards. If we could sedate them down in an hour and a half and get all that fixed, it was a much more efficient way of doing it for both us and for the patient. The practice really took off. We also did general anaesthetics, again with intravenous methohexitone.

I wasn't very keen on inhalation anaesthetics. I'd done, probably, about 30 or 40 as a dental student, and when I was in Chertsey, we had a general practitioner come in doing the GAs for us, and I didn't really particularly enjoy the sessions because I didn't feel comfortable with the patients in the state they were in under inhalation anaesthesia. Seeing how they did it at Walthamstow just changed my ideas completely about general anaesthetics. And so that's how we did it. In the whole of the time I was in Lincoln, I think I did only about 3 or 4 inhalational anaesthetics simply because I was unable to find a vein on the patient.

The practice took off and we worked ourselves silly; it was good fun.

Working with two nurses

In Walthamstow I'd always worked with two nurses. So, our philosophy was to always work with two nurses. Especially if you're doing sedations or anaesthesia, you need that number of staff with you.

I work a lot more efficiently if I'm not having to look for instruments, and I can sit with one nurse on my left side, and she's doing suction and the mixing, and another nurse on my right-hand side who's doing my burr changes and passing my instruments. And every procedure we would do in exactly the same way, with the same instruments, in the same order. When we were passing instruments between us, I'd always take all the instruments, I would never say I don't want one, they would give me the instrument. If I didn't want it, I would pass it straight back to them and we'd have the next one ready. We would have several hand pieces, so that I was never having to change the burr in a handpiece. Because while I'm doing some work, I might say to the nurse, I'd like an inverted cone next. So, she'd put an inverted cone into the handpiece. And it was those hand pieces that you just pull one off, pull another one on, she could do that and just hand it to me straight away. And so, I was working in a swifter more efficient way. And I wasn't getting frustrated with having to look around and do things that I didn't need to do.

As we developed the practice everybody worked with two nurses, including our associates. Later on in my career, when we actually sold the practice to a corporate, they tried to reduce the number of nurses we had. But when we did the agreement with them, I made sure that the complement of nurses would not be reduced. Because there was no way I was going to drop down to one nurse having been used to two and the efficiency that it gave me. One of the frustrations is the waiting time in between patients, you want to get on and keep moving and keep working. And so that allowed us to do that.

The dental health in Lincoln was pretty awful, because the place had been under-dentisted and people hadn't got treatment. So they were requiring a tremendous amount of work. We got investigated by the Dental Estimates Board, as it was called then. They sent us various charts about our prescribing patterns and said they needed to come and have a personal interview with us.

A dentist from the DEB visited the practice and said that he wanted to discuss our treatment patterns because he was concerned about the volume of crown and bridge work we were doing, and the number of extractions relative to root treatments. We were doing more root treatments than taking teeth out. And we said that if we could root treat a tooth and save it, we would tend to prefer to do that, and the patients seemed to like that as well. Anyway, he said that having come and seen what we were doing and how we were running the practice he could understand it.

But looking at all the statistics they'd got on us they could probably tell me how many times I went to the toilet in a day, there was so much breakdown of all the figures. In those days, you filled a lot of information into those FP17 forms, you had to mark everything down. So we had that investigation and we were never really bothered by them afterwards.

One of the big failings, I think, that the NHS dental service did was get rid of their Regional Dental Officers. We had a really nice RDO named David. He was doubly qualified and one day week was a demonstrator at Sheffield dental school. When he first came to the practice, he was a bit starchy, very formal. And, in retrospect, you can understand why because he had to keep that sort of relationship with you.

One of the first things he did was to say they had a dental surgery, not used for anything else other than the dental reference officer, to check out patients because that's what they used to do. They took a sample of your patients, check them and make sure that the standard of the work you're doing was okay, and that you were doing what you said you'd done. Also, if you'd applied for something that needed prior approval, and they wanted to examine the patient they would do it at that surgery. He said, 'This is silly, because we're keeping this surgery, and it's being used too infrequently to justify its existence.' So, he wrote to all the dentists as to whether they would allow him to do all the examinations in each surgery. So, your patients would be seen in your surgery, which of course, was nicer for the patients as well. He had a positive response from all the dentists and we could meet him face to face and he could also assess the practice condition and how it was managed. So, he used to come to the surgery.

After he'd been coming to us for about a year or so he became a lot more relaxed. We always treated him with utmost respect and asked his advice. He would come sometimes when we'd put in for approval of a big job, of something like eight crowns. And he might comment, 'yes, but the two upper sevens aren't looking too wonderful. Don't they need to be crowned at some stage?' I would often totally agree but comment that the DPB may be feeling that I was applying for too much. So, we had that nice working relationship. Then he started to refer patients to the practice from practitioners who had problems that they didn't feel that they could manage. So that was big kudos for us. That was lovely.

Rick and I started in 1975, then John Thorpe joined the practice as we had more patients than we could cope with.

Then in 1982 my original partner Rick Newton, decided to resign from dentistry and we then took on Martin Hargreaves; he joined us as an associate later on that year, Nigel Bourne then came and joined us as an associate and they both became partners, and that was a four-man partnership until I left in 2006, when the government introduced the dreadful new NHS contract for dentistry.

Anaesthesia.

I got heavily involved in SAAD, the Society for the Advancement of Anaesthesia in Dentistry. I became a member of the Council for a number of years, was membership secretary and helped to run the resuscitation courses at the BDA conferences.

In the later part of the 1990s, the Poswillo report on general anaesthesia came in and that was quite right. It was saying that people really should have a bit more formal training in dental anaesthesia rather than as it was in the initial SAAD days, where you went on the weekend course and you came away with a bag full of goodies and you could start plugging people in on Monday afternoon, if you wanted. And that was wrong.

The Poswillo report said training needed to be done and it needed to be move formalized. Eventually it got to the point where you could not give general anaesthetics in dental practice unless you were a consultant anaesthetist. And there was a sort of grandfather clause saying that if you were a dentist, or a doctor who worked with anaesthetics, but were not consultant, then you had to become registered with the Royal College of Anaesthetists as a non-consultant anaesthetist. And for that we had to do some training course.

That involved going into hospital to do anaesthetics, which was interesting and fun to do. But they weren't necessarily appropriate to the sort of anaesthetics we were doing in general practice, because we were doing short anaesthetics mostly for the extraction of teeth. Occasionally, we might do a bit of conservative dentistry but generally it was extracting teeth. I found it very interesting and we were very lucky in Lincoln to have Richard Thornton the anaesthetist, who was our mentor/examiner for it all. I went and did some anaesthetics with him. He did dental anaesthetics out in the community so I went and did some on his sessions. And there, I was using an inhalational anaesthetic using halothane, which was a technique I hadn't used very much, but interesting to do. But I still prefer doing intravenous anaesthesia.

Practice staff

We had a tremendously loyal staff, who would come to us at the age of 16, as one did in those days, and we would train them up and get them through the dental nursing exams. Some of them could actually do a lot more than just being a dental nurse and could perhaps be a hygienist and some of them went off, trained and came back to work as hygienists with us. Other members of staff would get married and have kids, and then come back and work part time with us and then full time again once the kids were of an age that they could do that. We would very often keep staff for a long time. I had the same two nurses for close to 28 years. I still see a lot of the staff that used to be working with and it's delight to see him.

Remuneration, fee per item-of-service

We were paid a fee for each item we did. So it was so much for an examination, for bitewings, a scale and polish, and an occlusal amalgam, all separate fees. An MO on a molar would be one and if it had an extension on it, that would be a separate fee. It was a really complicated system that should have been sorted out with not so many fees. The government constantly fiddled around with the patient's charges. We had some weird ones, like the patient pays the full cost of the treatment, up to £17. And then 40% of the cost of treatment after that. They weren't designed to encourage people to come regularly, in my mind.

So, in 1998 the fee for an examination was £5.65. If you did an extensive examination and report that included a full periodontal charting, you've got £8. An extraction of one tooth was £5.65. So that obviously encouraged people not to take teeth out.

You can see the complexities of all the things you had to work out, but we were computerized by 1992 so then it became relatively easy to do, but if it was done by hand with a nurse looking through charts to work out the different fees, it was difficult.

In the early 1990s they brought in registration so that you got paid a fee for having a patient on your books, because prior to that, and then subsequent, patients were not actually registered with you. They came for a course of treatment. Basically, you were setting up and going into a contract with that patient for that course of treatment with a third party, the health service, making their contribution. Then in the early 1990s they came in with a registration and you got paid a fixed amount. And if they needed treatment, you got a further enhancement.

And that was crazy. We pointed out when they brought out the proposals that if I saw a kid that needed five fillings, I would get the appropriate fee for doing that amount of work. But if I referred that child to another dentist, they would also get the same fee again, that I had received, while I still kept the fee. So, it could be paid twice. And that was not fair on the finances of the health service. It was nuts. And there were lots of dentists who were just seeing kids, getting the fee, and referring them on to somewhere else. Really mad!

Then the government realized that too much money was being spent so they cut the fees by a gross figure of 7%. Our practice expenses were over 60% per dentist. So, the 7% was coming off, about 35%, a much greater proportion of our income was going that way. And that was one of the big surges for people to go private.

That was in 1992. I carried on seeing all my health service patients. I had quite a large list, over 4000 patients on the health service. But at that point, I stopped taking on completely new families for health service treatment; I would see extended members of the family groups. But I was still seeing loads and loads of patients, and it was too big; it was becoming unmanageable.

At that time, I had a private list of only about 300 to 400. And those were only because people who wanted to come privately, not because I said that's the only way I would treat them. I wasn't terribly keen on some of the insurance schemes like Denplan. I did have some Denplan patients, but I never sold it. It was not something I necessarily recommended to people. But if they came to me and said they wanted to do it, I would talk them through what I thought the prosthetics and conservative dentistry they needed was, then I would happily take them on as I felt I had put them in a position of them given me 'informed consent'.

So, then any new people that really wanted to see me, then I would see them privately. But I still believed in trying to do as much as I could to people under the health service.

The contract of 2006 was another spur for lots of dentists to leave the health service and go fully private. Looking at the 'Admore' FP 17 guide card for April 2000 an extraction was £6.05 and if they had a general anaesthetic, that was an additional £19.36. We carried on doing GAs, and we knew they were something that it was costing us to do, but we felt it was the right thing to do for our patients.

At one point, I did take referrals from other dentists for GAs, but then I stopped doing that. I saw the patients and spoke to them and sometimes the dentists were just trying to get rid of what might be considered by them to be a difficult extraction. So they would say to the patient that they probably needed to go to sleep to have the tooth taken out. And yet, I would see them and tell them that they had a choice. If they were happy I could do it under local anaesthetic. And they would often say they had been told it needed a general anaesthetic but that they were quite happy to have a local anaesthetic. I felt that, as in the hospital service, that referral service can act as a dumping ground of people who the dentists who don't want.

Partnership

Our partnership was worked on the basis of expense sharing. We took the gross expenses of the practice and shared it equally amongst ourselves. We separated out laboratory fees and each paid his own laboratory fees. We changed it a little bit after a number of years because two of my colleagues were doing a tremendous amount of orthodontic work, a lot of fixed work.

So, all the expenses were shared equally. Another thing was the hygienist fees; we separated out the hygienist fees, otherwise, one guy sending a lot of patients to the hygienist would be getting unfairly subsidized by a guy who perhaps didn't send her so many patients.

We had associates in my earlier years. We didn't pay the 50% which is what most people did; we paid 45%. The reason it was 45% was because we gave associates two nurses and opportunities to use more than one surgery. They could therefore maximize their income by being more efficient and providing those services was a greater charge on us. We didn't have any dentists complain about that, because they could see when they got the actual figures that they were actually earning very good income.

Overall, our practice expenses were about 60%, so perhaps a dentist would be better off as an associate than as a partner. In my unofficial role as a dental advisor to some colleagues, when they come and tell me what their associates are grossing, I've said 'you cannot afford this' and one very good friend of ours had three associates working for him and he couldn't understand why he was taking home less money than when he worked on his own. Until we talked through it and I said 'well, the extra expenses you're paying for your associates means you're actually subsidising them'.

New contract of 2006

Retirement is a word I no longer use for that period because I retired from the practice that I built up when the new contract was coming in. I was probably getting a little bit jaded myself and tired; it had been a busy practicing life. And when the new contract was proposed, I was quite heavily involved in dental politics. I'd been sitting on the LDC,[99] and been dental advisor to regions and sitting on service committees, and I always kept myself well aware of what was going on. When the new contract came out, I read what it was proposing, and I couldn't see that it was right for the dentists or patients, and sadly it has proven to be true.

One of my partners said to me that I was looking at it completely the wrong way. I was looking at it as a contract that should be fair to people. And it was not, it was all about control so that they could limit the expenditure from the health service and control what we were doing and where we practised. Because up until that point, with a fee per item, you could just keep putting in claim after claim and they would meet them. I could see it from a treasury point of view, they couldn't say, our budget for this year is going to be X million on dentistry, because it was an open-ended contract with us making as many claims as we wanted. They could estimate it, and with the amount of evidence they'd had, they could get it reasonably accurate. But the new contract meant that they could come in and they could say exactly how much they were going to be putting out in a year.

They took a 12-month period of what you'd done, what you'd grossed in fees, and then they could work out what your 'Units of Dental Activity' would be financed. One unit you'd get for doing examination, X rays and scale and polishes, then it's been three units if you did the examinations and any other dentistry that didn't involve laboratory work. So, my UDA was going to be estimated about 20 pounds. And Nigel, working next door and John and Martin, we all had different values of units of dental activity. So, I would get those 20 pounds for doing one UDA. But for three UDAs, I'd get approximately £60. But I'd have to do whatever needed to be done that didn't involve the laboratory work. If I took a new patient on and that new patient needed extensive periodontal work, a molar root treatment and four or five fillings it was still £60. That can't be done for £60.

At the end of the day, dentists are running a business and if that business does not make any profit, then the business folds, and you have

---

[99] Local Dental Committee.

no dentistry. If you want to have a successful dental practice, it has to be financially viable. I could not see under this system how it was going to be financially sound and I didn't think it was fair. So, I decided that it was probably time for me to leave general practice which I did on the 31st of March 2006. So, on the April Fool's Day, the next day, the new contract was brought in.

Local Dental Committee

For the vast majority of time I was on the LDC it was a social club, but it was nowhere near the amount of involvement that the present LDC have with the Health Service, and the amount of work they do. We were advising, we did service committees, and we would be advising on areas where there was poor dental coverage and how we might be able to encourage more dentists to go there.

The LDC was concerned about single handed dental practitioners, working on their own. I feel that working on your own all the time is not a satisfactory way to practise. We tried to make contact with as many of those chaps as we could just to get them to come along and be involved in things like the BDA meetings where they could meet with people who understand the stresses of their job; because nobody understands the stresses of a particular job unless they actually work it.

People underestimate, I think, the stress of doing dentistry in a general practice, where you're seeing people, the majority of whom don't want to be there. And how you have to alter your behaviour from a five-year-old child to a 65-year-old lady to a 17-year-old girl and backwards and forwards throughout the day, you're changing your behaviour. And you are trying to do intricate work on people in difficult situations.

The British Dental Association

When I first came to Lincoln, the BDA meetings were held out at Market Rasen, which I know is only about 25 miles away, in the Gordon Arms. John Bayes[100] was brought up there because his father had run the pub many years ago and we had our meetings there. We'd have a back room in the pub, dried up sandwiches and then a speaker would come. I felt it was not the right way for us to be having professional meetings. So I, with the then maxillofacial surgeon, Ian Alexander, set up the Lincoln BDA and that has been extremely successful.

---

[100] See chapter 12.

We got admonished a little bit by the BDA in our early years, because they said we should not be inviting national or international speakers to our meetings, because we might get a poor turnout and that wouldn't be good for the BDA. But we were getting 25 people coming along to dine and now another dozen or 15 come along for the speaker afterwards. We had never experienced anything from our speakers other than that they really liked coming to our meetings. And they said one of the lovely things they find about coming to the Lincoln section is there doesn't seem to be any backbiting. Everybody seems to be so friendly to each other.

Diploma in General Dental Practice.

I got involved with some regional boards as well. One of the interesting ones was when the they set up the Diploma in General Dental Practice at the Royal College of Surgeons, DGDP; later they changed it to the MFGDP.[101] John Bayes, a good friend, was invited to go on the Regional Board for it. He came to me as he didn't want to do it and asked me if I would, which I agreed to do.

I went along and, at the first meeting I went to, it came up in conversation that they'd all been given an honorary diploma, and I hadn't got one. They said they'd get me one. but I didn't want it unless I'd earned it. I also thought it would be valuable if we had one person on the board that had actually done the exam, which they thought was a bit weird.

So, I did that and did it in conjunction with Nigel Bourne, one of my partners, and we worked together on it and that was hard work because it covered absolutely everything from running your business to the clinical aspects of dentistry. I can remember going to my viva, there were two dentists there and they started firing questions at me. The questions were going from employment law to antibiotic prophylaxis or something, backwards and forwards and they started getting faster and faster as I was trying to keep up with them. When I finished, I went off and was just completely bombed out.

I was very pleased to get it. If I hadn't, I would have come off the board immediately. That also was a pleasure for me, because when I first graduated, I didn't go to any graduation ceremonies so when I got my diploma, it was a joy to be able to take my mother up to the formal ceremony at Royal College of Surgeons. That was a delight.

---

[101] Member of the Faculty of General Dental Practice.

19. Barry Cockcroft

General Dental Practitioner who became involved in local and then national dental politics. After joining a pilot scheme for capitation payments in general practice he was asked to help promote it and subsequently to become deputy Chief Dental Officer for England. Later as Chief Dental Officer he oversaw the introduction of two new dental schools, a school for dental therapists, the publication of the first edition of 'Delivering Better Oral Health' and the introduction of the 2006 dental contract which introduced local commissioning for dentistry. He spoke to me at his home in 2023 about this and other issues during his time as CDO.

******

Dental School

It was always my ambition to be a veterinary surgeon and so my chosen A levels were biology, physics and chemistry. But in my last school year I spent a few days with a vet in Bolton, and he was totally disillusioned, particularly with putting down healthy animals that he could save, but were just inconvenient. So I went completely off it.

I got my A levels and was offered a place to do veterinary medicine, turned it down and decided to take a year off.

I took a year off, took a gap year, in 1968/69 and worked in a foundry in Bolton. It was very hard, dirty, poorly paid and dangerous. And that actually made me more aware of how privileged I was to have a job that you could actually enjoy. I was never ever bored as a dentist.

Birmingham was a great place to study dentistry. There were some fantastic people who really formed me. The staff were great, but two people particularly inspired me. Ivor Whitehead, who was a really down to earth guy and Don Glenwright, who was head of Periodontology and taught us all about professionalism.

I won the surgery and anaesthesia prize at Birmingham and my ambition was to be a maxillofacial surgeon. So I got a job at Coventry in the Oral and Maxillofacial Surgery department, or the Dental Department as it was called at the time. It was orthodontics and oral surgery but also A & E and follow up. Halfway through that year, it became obvious that to become a maxillofacial surgeon I'd need to go back to university and do a medical degree. I got married in August of that year and I wasn't willing to put my wife through the rigours of travelling around the country getting jobs and being a student for another five years. So I packed that up and went to work in general practice, which actually I thoroughly enjoyed.

General Practice

At first, starting in 1975, I was three years in a lovely practice in Coventry; it was before vocational training started. The principal of the practice, John Mander, was wonderful so it was a bit like being in a vocational training practice.

John was never the sort of person who was going to have a partner; he was always going to be the person in charge and I wanted to join a practice where I could be a partner. So I applied for an associate posting in Rugby. I looked around the practice, which was a little old-fashioned, and pointed this out to the partners. They said that they wanted someone to modernise.

I was lucky because there was a shortage of associates then so an associate could really pick and choose where they went. There was a boiling water steriliser in each surgery and where I came from, we had autoclaves. But I liked this practice and I liked the town and I looked around and said that I would join them on condition that was an autoclave in each surgery and they quickly agreed to that.

Then I just brought a bit of what you might call modern thinking to the practice, and we changed a lot of things. There was an in-house laboratory and I said that I thought it would be better contracting out the technical work and putting in another surgery because there was a huge demand and we couldn't treat all the people we wanted to treat. So we closed the laboratory and installed another surgery. We got an OPG machine and started sending our nurses on training courses and upskilling them as much as we could. It was difficult at the time because there was no statutory registration for dental nurses. We got a hygienist which they hadn't had before.

I stayed there from 1979 until I went to work at the Department of Health in 2002. Even then I carried on working Saturday mornings for two years until 2004, because I just enjoyed it. I got very close to my patients; they were friends.

We had a very successful practice. The problem was, by 2002 when I got offered the job at the Department of Health, I'd been seeing my patients there for 20 years, and they were almost all disease free. I could spend a whole day in the practice not seeing a carious lesion. Financially it worked, but with regular patients it was not challenging clinically. It wasn't boring because I liked the people, but I just needed more of a challenge. When I went to the Department, I took a drop in earnings of 30,000 pounds. But it wasn't clinically challenging by the time I'd left, so the offer came at just the right time.[102]

First involvement in dental politics

In 1980 when I became a partner, my partners said the Local Dental Committee wanted somebody to join them, and as we were the biggest practice in Rugby, they thought it should be one of us and suggested me; I was the youngest person in the practice. So I joined the Warwickshire Local Dental Committee and later became secretary and subsequently chairman.

Then I got elected to the General Dental Service Committee, GDSC, of the British Dental Association representing Coventry, Warwickshire and Solihull. The GDSC negotiated with the government; they represented at a national level.

So I moved from local to national and learned a lot at the BDA and met some lovely people there and got to meet people at the Department of Health and to understand how the system worked. There were some great people at the BDA and there were some other people who were less than well motivated in terms of the NHS. But that's the real world, and you have to learn how that works.

When I went to the GDSC I started to understand the problems that people faced. There had been a referendum on a new contract and various things that were introduced in 1990. And the referendum had voted to reject it, and then the BDA accepted it.[103] That was the first attempt at paying a capitation payment. It had been a great success, so successful that the commitment payments budget was overspent. And

---

[102] Barry worked in general dental practice for 27 years.
[103] The General Dental Services Committee of the BDA had negotiated the contract which brought in capitation, continuing care and prevention. A conference of Local Dental Committees had voted in favour but when it was put to a referendum only 38% voted to accept. The GDSC ignored that, the excuse was that the resistance was from only some geographical areas, particularly London which wanted to stay with the item-of-service payment system. See: British Dental Journal July 21 1990 Vol 169 (2) P33.

that caused all sorts of grief, because the government cut the fees in 1992. That started off the growth in private practice and the exodus away from the NHS. And when people went away from the NHS, there was nothing the NHS could do to replace them because there was no local health budget.

The fee cut had been traumatic for me in practice and such a learning experience. We were a profit-sharing practice. So we partners drew out the same amount from the practice, each partner every year, and we had a reconciliation at the end of the year. We went to see our accountant, and it was worse because the doctors and dentists review body had recommended an increase of, I think it was, 11%. But when they took into account earnings and stuff like that, it ended up being a fee cut of 7%, and we were not prepared for this. We saw our accountant; we had looked at his figures, and asked why is this bottom figure in brackets? And were told that it was because, taking into account our drawings, we had made a loss that year.

That came as a shock to us and a shock that he hadn't told us already. So we looked at everything and changed lots of things. My wife started doing the wages for the staff, we centralised ordering and we started to make ourselves more efficient.

But a lot of people weren't willing to do that. And that really kick-started Denplan. They came to Rugby and we had a big meeting at the golf club. They told us that if we left the NHS and went into Denplan, the NHS couldn't do anything about it. 50% of our patients would stay with us, we would earn the same amount of money and we would be doing less work because we'd only be seeing 50% of the patients. Isn't that great? And we asked what about the other 50% of our patients who can't afford it? And they said, 'Well, that's somebody else's problem.' We were not ready to do that, so we said no.

After the fee cut in 1992, there was the Bloomfield report, and we had a special General Dental Services Committee meeting.[104] We had committees: there was a Fee Scale Committee, which negotiated changes to the fee scale, and we had a Stats. and Regs. Committee, which

---

[104] Fundamental Review of Dental Remuneration. Report of Sir Kenneth Bloomfield KCB. 1992. Among its 49 recommendations it suggested: ' In the longer term, consideration needs to be given to more radical options...such as re-defining the ambit of NHS dentistry, in terms of categories of treatments, categories of patients or both; moving to a more locally-sensitive or even devolved system of administration; and replacing a single remuneration system with a range of options which could be adapted to local use.

negotiated on changes to regulations. There was a Superannuation Committee, which discussed the NHS pension and how it related to dentists. And there was an Executive Committee, which met with people at the top of dentistry and the government to talk about the future. But I thought it was very much lip-service because the government were just going to do what they were going to do anyway.

Later, when I went to work at the Department of Health in 2002, I met people who were there when the fee cut was made and I now know that the dental people within the Department of Health told the Treasury people that this would be disastrous for the NHS, but all they were interested in was the money. And they insisted on the fee cut, and that was a real challenge.

Pilot for Personal Dental Service

In 1997, at the fag end of the Tory government they introduced something called Personal Dental Services pilots, which was an opportunity to get away from item-of-service payment. I wanted to do this so in our practice we piloted a system which was based on adult capitation. The government thought this was doable but the dental profession was completely sceptical. We actually made it work in our practice and two other practices in the town.

There were lots of options for how it could work, but it had to stick with primary legislation, and so the patients' charging system had to stay the same, it was not allowed to have a different charging system.

We were just paid a regular monthly sum for each patient we had on our books, no matter what we did for them. And it worked for us, most of our patients were dentally fit. If we got a new patient, we would make them dentally fit using the item-of-service based system, so that we weren't taking on somebody with a massive need for a relatively low payment.

Then I got involved centrally. Everybody hated item-of-service payment at the time. Dentistry has always complained about the system of payment, which had never changed. The first reporting into the inappropriate dental systems was the Tattersall report in the mid- 1960s, and then the Bloomfield report in 1992.[105]

Then Margaret Seward,[106] who was my mentor for a long time, asked me to go round and explain to dentists how the capitation system works. So I did. Then she said, 'This needs to happen. We're going to do this, a policy change.' This led to the policy document 'Options for Change' which was published in 2002.[107]

Margaret asked me if I would write the section on service delivery. 'Systems of delivery of dental care', was the bit I wrote. We met as a group and I had a minder, Tony Jenner, who then was a consultant in public health in Liverpool, in the Strategic Health Authority. They wanted to make sure that the people who led the three working groups didn't go off piste. Tony Jenner was brilliant and we became great friends. When I became deputy Chief Dental Officer Tony became head of Quality and Standards at the Department of Health, and when I became CDO, we just moved Tony up to be my deputy.

Then Dame Margaret took me out for dinner and said that they were going to create a job for me, in London, called Deputy Chief Dental Officer. There had never been one before but it was to be created for me although I would have to apply and go through the process. So having written for the document, I didn't expect 18 months later to be working at the Department of Health.

Margaret Seward was not statutorily appointed at Chief Dental Officer so she could only be appointed for two years. They went through the appointment process to replace her and Raman Bedi was appointed. But they knew that they wanted to take forward Options for Change and the Minister responsible for dentistry was Lord Philip Hunt, who is now the president of the British Fluoridation Society, somebody I know well. Margaret had explained to Philip that Options for Change needed to be

---

[105] Methods of Remuneration. Report of Committee under chairmanship of W. R. Tattersall. It reported in 1964. Among its recommendations were: 'That the General Dental Services Committee consider the introduction in due course of a system of remuneration for the general dental services based on capitation fess for the routine maintenance of dental fitness plus fees by scale for dentures and more complex items of treatment.' It was published in the British Dental Journal. 117 (8) 331-346 Oct 20 1964.

[106] Dame Margaret was Chief Dental Officer from 2000 to 2002.

[107] NHS Dentistry: Options for Change was published in August 2002. Barry was Vice Chairman of the General Dental Services of the Committee of the British Dental Association at that time. Margaret Seward had appointed him as the Chairman of the Task Group for the 'systems of delivery of dental care' part of the report which concluded that the best way to deliver dental care was to separate dentists' income from individual treatments and proposed different options of this might be achieved.

implemented and that they needed a deputy, who knew about primary care dentistry, to lead the introduction for new system. So they created this new post and I came in as Deputy Chief Dental Officer to Raman.

Later, when Raman left, they made me Acting Chief Dental Officer. The thing that brought it about was piloting PDS nationwide before the transition to the new contract in 2006. I told them it was the wrong thing to do, patients' charge revenue would fall, that they wouldn't be able to maintain it and it would just mess up the whole system, which it did. And when Raman left, somebody asked why didn't anybody say that this was a disaster. And David Hewlett, who was head of the dental division at the Department of Health said: 'actually, Barry said this would be a disaster'. And that got me the job as acting CDO in February 2005, although the outside world wasn't told until a bit later, and I stayed there until 2015, and saw through the change in 2006.[108]

But I didn't have the essential criteria to be appointed as Chief Dental Officer, so they got around that by changing the essential criteria, because the essential criteria for the job meant that a general practitioner could never be CDO; you needed to have a list of publications and postgraduate qualifications. The person who had been CDO had always been an academic or somebody from the services. And, you know, primary care dentistry provides 96% of the service and academia provides about 4%, but takes 20% of the money. So they changed the essential criteria so that a general practitioner could be become CDO. There has never been a CDO who was a general practitioner before me and there hasn't been one since.

Item-of-service payment

People who are saying fee for item-of-service was the best way never worked in it. And it caused immense damage to public health. Basically, the idea that the more you drill, the more you get paid was complete anathema to me. Anybody of my age knows what an Australian trench is; it was an amalgam that runs from the mesial of the eight to the distal of the four all amalgam, done in every quadrant. It earned a fantastic amount of money and damaged the teeth tremendously.

I went for an interview in a practice not far from here before I came to Rugby where I was told that the practice never did occlusal fillings. If

---

[108] Barry became Deputy Chief Dental Officer for England in November 2002, acting Chief Dental Officer in October 2005 and Chief Dental Officer from July 2006 to 2015.

it was an occlusal it had to be an MO, DO or an MOD because you got paid more for doing that.

Item-of-service payment, although easy to administer, had awful oral health implications. And the BDA were manically opposed to item-of-service; they used to call it the item-of-service treadmill. Prevention doesn't fit into item-of-service payment. But having said that, somebody once said to me, there's no good way of paying dentists but the three worst are item-of-service, capitation and a salary. Basically, you've got to rely on the dentist to be professional and do the right thing for the patients. And I always believe that the vast majority of people will do that.

The first report into the inappropriateness of item-of-service was the Tattersall report in 1964. And there was the Bloomfield report in 1992 and then Options for Change. Although the BDA were opposed to item-of-service they never said what they would put in place, and I strongly believe that the right way to pay dentists is a system of weighted capitation, which is what I'd done in Rugby, and which Margaret liked.

And of course, the whole thing has changed and oral health has changed. When I graduated 70% of kids had caries. Now over 80% of kids are caries free so item-of-service payment doesn't work in a situation where the disease levels are falling. For when I graduated in 1973, 40% of the adult population were edentulous. That compared appallingly with the rest of Europe. It doesn't mean our oral health was worse; it just means that the item-of-service payment-based system which, when I graduated, paid a fortune for doing full clearances and fitting full dentures for people. That was the wrong thing to do, but the system incentivized that.

When I first went to work in John's practice in Coventry in 1975, the first Thursday afternoon was denture afternoon. There were all these people booked in to have inspections and full clearances. And I examined them and I said they didn't all need a full clearance. I would sort them out and only remove the carious teeth and the ones that were periodontally unsavable. And some of them accepted it and some of them didn't. John was furious. He said 'Have any idea how much money we get for doing that?' And I said, 'Well, I'm not going to do it if it's not the right thing.'

And the reason our country had more edentulousness was that we had a national health service introduced in 1948, so that the general public could actually afford dental treatment, whereas there was no NHS in

Europe. So elsewhere people retained their grotty periodontally involved carious teeth to some degree, but didn't end up edentulous. And if you look at it now, the number of people who are edentulous is very low, single figures, less than 5%, I think.

If people now are saying we want item-of-service payment, they need to speak to some of the people who worked in item-of-service 30 years ago. The Schanschiff[109] report illustrated the downside of item-of-service, that dentists would drill unnecessarily. The report focused on the people who were over treating on item-of-service to earn large amounts of money. That happened, but it was a small number of people. That's what Schanschiff was about; it didn't reflect well on the profession. It didn't represent the majority of the profession. The majority of the profession was, and still is, working damn hard to do a good job for their patients.

I had a personal experience with this when I was working in hospital after graduating. I locumed on my afternoon off because I was short of money, in a practice locally. I worked on a day book, wrote in the daybook what I'd done and then they would submit the forms with one of the principals' names on. One day I finished, had written the day book and my nurse had put the details on the FP17 forms. I went to my car but returned because I had left my shopping in the surgery. The principal was in the surgery, going through these FP17s. And he was adding a scale and polish and two bitewings to every form. But they hadn't had a scale and polish and two bitewings, and that was total abuse of the system. I asked what he was doing and he just said we should claim this because there's no way they can check, and we get more money. So I left that day and never went back.

Chief Dental Officer

The role of Chief Dental Officer has changed a bit, because when I joined, I was part of the Department of Health. There was no NHS England. It was the Department of Health so the people who ran the NHS reported directly back to the Secretary of State. Later, in 2010, they set up NHS England, which separated from the Department of Health. My job was NHS; but it was a given, and it was in my job specification that I would also advise on all dental issues. So I covered all things related to dentistry, some which you'd expect, and so much you wouldn't expect.

---

[109] Report of the Committee of Enquiry into Unnecessary Dental Treatment. HMSO 1986.

It was not just the NHS. I spent a lot of time going backwards and forwards to Brussels to get the European Union regulations on tooth whitening changed. When I started, the European Union legislation said that the amount of hydrogen peroxide you could use in a tooth whitening process product was 0.1% which actually doesn't work; it is not effective. And we were trying to change the concentration, I think, to 1%, which I think is effective.

It involved NHS contracts that had nothing to do with private contracts, but things like the Care Quality Commission and decontamination standards; all these things were just as applicable to the private sector as they are to the NHS. So I covered a whole range of things. And I worked with other government departments. I worked on Professional Regulation, because when I started, I was an associate member of the General Dental Council, so I sat on that GDC, but I didn't vote. But the GDC is not within the remit of the Chief Dental Officer; it's controlled by something called Professional Regulation Department. But when they were discussing the GDC, they would always ask me to attend.

At one point, when the GDC was particularly dysfunctional, there was quite a lot of pressure and ministers were minded to abolish it. And we had an offer from the General Medical Council that they would take the GDC and make it a subcommittee of the General Medical Council. I went to a lot of quite high-powered meetings and spoke vehemently against it. I did not want to be the Chief Dental Officer at a time when the General Dental Council was abolished.

Mercury in crematoria

One issue I had to deal with was crematoria. They were introducing scrubbers in the chimneys of crematoria. And years ago, when people died, they were edentulous and it wasn't a big issue. But now older people are dentate with multiple restorations, and they were looking to provide information as to what the specification for scrubbers should be in crematoria. We had to work out how many filled teeth the average person who died had, what the weight of the filling was, therefore, how much mercury was potentially being given into the atmosphere by cremating these people with multiple restorations. It was the sort of thing that you could never in your wildest dreams imagine somebody would ask you. When you work in the department, you do get asked the most bizarre things. Sometimes it was quite interesting, sometimes quite challenging.

Decontamination

Another issue was decontamination. In 2010 there was an attempt to get a new minister to remove me because I was introducing HTM [Health Technical Memorandum] 01-05, which they didn't like, and the Care Quality Commission. Dame Margaret had been keeping me informed of what was going on and, in the end, it just reinforced my position with the Minister.

HTM 01-05 was absolutely necessary.[110] All it did was collate all the guidance that was already there. At the time, BSE [Bovine Spongiform Encephalopathy] was a big issue, and there was something called the Spongiform Encephalopathy Advisory Committee, SEAC, who were convinced that dentistry was spreading CJD [Creutzfeldt-Jakob disease]. There was no evidence to support that, and they wanted all dental instruments to be single use. It would have obliterated dentistry. So I said that they couldn't do that and there was no evidence to support what they wanted. In dentistry we are used to using decontamination equipment. But there were articles published in the BDJ showing blood in the hinges of forceps after autoclaving which rather undermined my argument.

So I finally came to an agreement with SEAC which said, if we can produce agreed guidance on decontamination will you stop pushing to have dental instruments – which are not owned by the NHS but by dentists – to make them single use? So HTM 01-05 effectively avoided SEAC pursuing single-use dental instruments as advice to the Government. Although there was nothing new in it, it was just best practice made clear.

Decontamination in dentistry is quite a challenge because areas such as the abdomen or brain are sterile, the mouth is a mucky area. I remember going to an Infection Protection Society meeting at Warwick University and saying that dental instruments do not need to be sterile, and there was a sharp intake of breath. I said dental instruments need to have been sterilised after they were used on one patient and stored appropriately before being used again. The mouth is full of bugs. So it's about preventing cross infection, it's not about sterile instruments; the moment you start to use a dental instrument, it is not sterile.

---

[110] HTM 01-05, Decontamination: Health Technical Memorandum 01-05 – Decontamination in primary care dental practices. It was published by the Department of Health in 2013. It gave guidance on cleaning, disinfection and sterilizing reusable dental equipment.

It was a really difficult time. The first draft of HTM 01-05 said that each dental surgery should have positive pressure, so that when you opened the door, the air flows out. It was total bollocks. And one of the few people I sacked was a guy who wrote the first draft. Saying sacked is not quite right, I didn't have the power to sack him, but I told his boss that he had come back with a second draft, which was, again, totally unacceptable and I wanted him off my team. And they removed him. HTML 01-05 is actually a very sensible document. There was nothing new in it. It was just pulling together everything that was already there.

The dental profession was dead against it, because at the time that BDA had a policy being against anything that government did, and they were causing quite a riot about the Care Quality Commission, as well.

New dental contract 2006

People don't understand how long it takes to initiate legislation. One of the things I'd said in Options for Change was that there must be no big bang; we must do it in consultation with the profession.

I started at the Department of Health on November 4th 2002 at nine o'clock. At twenty past nine the head of the dental division came into the office and said 'hello Barry' and I detected a bit of nervousness, and he said that we were going to implement Option for Change in April 2005. I said that we couldn't do that as it was only two years away and there must be no big bang. He said we've been told that we cannot phase it in. It had to happen on one day because you couldn't take a non-cash limited budget, make it a cash limited budget, and phase it in. It's just not possible financially.

So in my job at the department I was relaxed for about 20 minutes. And I remember coming home that night. My flat wasn't ready, so I was staying in a hotel in London and the first big decision I had to make as Deputy Chief Dental Officer was whether, having found out that this was going to happen suddenly, I'd stick it out and see it through.

Access to dental care was going down the pan at the time. Tony Blair had said, in the Labour Party Conference in 1999, that everybody should be able to see an NHS dentist just by calling NHS Direct. And, without commissioning, that could never be met. And that's what caused the legislation to be started. Blair said, 'I want to control NHS dentistry'. And that's what local commissioning does, or what it's meant to do if it's adequately funded and resourced through the workforce. So that's why the plan for legislation was already in place before I started, which came as a bit of a shock on the day.

We thought the GP contract was going to be done in 2004 and we would follow the next year, 2005. And because they would have done the GPs, it would make it much easier for us. But it made it much more difficult because they'd given the doctors a whole load more money for doing less work, and got grief. A perfect storm. And then they started reorganising the Primary Care Trusts and reduced them down from 311 to 150, which was a nightmare. And eventually they said, 'look, we will delay it. We won't introduce it in April 2005; we will introduce it in April 2006', which is when it actually happened.

The legislation brought in control and local budgets. Access was disastrous in the late 90s, and early 2000s, because the government had cut the fees for item-of-service. There were queues around the block in Scarborough, and there were areas of the country where there was no access at all because the dentists controlled access. That's why local commissioning was introduced in 2006.

But we wanted another currency for the contract. And so we set up a working group, which was three people from the Department of Health and three people from the BDA, an ad hoc working group. And that working group came back and said, the right way to remunerate was on weighted courses of treatment. They recommended a simple course of treatment, a more complex course of treatment, and then a very complex course of treatment. So that ad hoc working group came up with a concept which became a Unit of Dental Activity. I was not part of that working group, and so I find it a bit narking when people say UDAs were my idea, which they weren't. But the legislation and contract is incredibly flexible

The principal aim of the new contract was to get rid of the item-of-service payment system and to get local commissioning and therefore control. It did controlled spending, but upwards.

We spent more money and we brought in more people so the spend went up. Since 1992, and the fee cut access had been going down steadily, because it was purely controlled by the dentist, the government could do nothing about it. And that was in Options for Change, how could we change it and I said without commissioning, you can't control it. Or you'd have to spend ridiculous amounts of money to incentivize people, which the finance people would never have had. So the introduction of local commissioning, came out of Options for Change. But I wasn't at the Department of Health then and the policy decision to actually implement it was taken before I got to the Department of Health.

We piloted capitation before 2006 in Personal Dental Service pilots. We just told people to put all their patients on this and they would be paid so much per month for each patient. We asked them to stick with it until 2006. And dentists liked that.

But some took the mickey and didn't see their patients at all. Some people were just working two or three days a week, keeping their existing patients who were dentally fit, who didn't need a recall, extending their recall intervals and not filling the space. It was a real challenge at the time. If somebody came and they needed a lot of treatment they just didn't take them on. There was no incentive to take on new patients whatsoever. And that's a simple capitation-based system.

The first pilot was not weighted capitation, it was just pure capitation. We introduced weighted capitation later on because we realised that there'd be some people who were more at risk. There was a full risk assessment. Each patient had to be risk assessed and then assigned to a risk register. So the capitation payment was higher for people who were high risk. There is no risk assessment in the UDA system. The UDA system is just weighted items of service really.

You can do prevention on a capitation basis and get rid of routine six monthly recalls for the vast majority of people who don't need them. But the problem is that the patients' charge revenue is linked to item-of-service. So in our pilot patients' revenue fell by about 30% because we were not doing scaling and polishing routinely if people didn't need them and we weren't doing bitewing radiography every six months because people didn't need it. And patients' charge revenue raises about 900 million pounds a year so a drop of 30%, 300 million pounds. There was a big fight with government finance people, because of the loss of patients' charge revenue.

But what we should have done was to introduce a transitional period so that people who were already being seen regularly went straight in, so you didn't have to put people who had been seen for 20 years through a full risk assessment, which took 20 minutes. So access actually dropped when the pilots started but we could have resolved that with more work. The patients liked it and there was more prevention. But the government were not willing to go down a capitation route at that time.

Item-of-services payment in the wrong hands can be very damaging. If you overprescribe that damage is there for life. Fillings never get smaller; every time they're replaced, they get bigger. But I liked capitation because the way a capitation based system is abused is under prescription of treatment. And I used to say to people that if you see under treatment, you can put it right.

When we set up our pilot, we had someone from Denplan on the steering group. Denplan is capitation based. And they had a department which mediated when patients moved from one area to another and the new dentist said 'oh you need six fillings' and they'd been not been done at the previous practice because they'd been paid on capitation; they'd been under treated. But there is no system that's not abusable.

The BDA did a survey about how many dentists would sign up to this new contract and their survey said that 97% of dentists would reject this new contract. I remember going to see Rosie Winterton the minister. And she said 'Barry, the BDA say that 97% of dentists will reject the NHS contract'. I said, 'That won't happen; they can't afford to, most of them. They'd lose their pension.' And in the end, we lost 3% of service over April 2006; that was about 1000 dentists.

Most of the dentists who turned it down had only got a small NHS commitment. And that was very silly because if you've got a very small NHS commitment you should hang on to it because it dynamizes your pension.

So the contract followed on from Options for Change. It implemented local commissioning, which was what Options for Change said because that gave the NHS control. We then provided extra money and put money into areas where there previously had been no NHS dentistry. It also meant that, for example, if my practice which had a budget of about a million pounds prior to 2006 left the NHS and had gone completely private, that million pounds would have just gone back into the Treasury and been spent on something else. After 2006, that million pounds goes back into the local NHS budget, and they could go to tender, and somebody else could tender for a contract using that million pounds and people did. So it completely changed the dynamic of dentistry.

When I started at the Department of Health, I asked what the budget was the previous year and it was 1.7 billion; within four years, it was 3 billion. We put a lot of extra money in. There were areas of the country which were completely without NHS dentistry. The spend had been going down, because dentists were pulling away from the NHS, and the NHS couldn't do anything about it, it had no control. Dentists control access, and that's what 2006 stopped.

There is a large amount of flexibility in the legislation which is not being used. In the northeast they are awash with money at the moment because there is not enough workforce to deliver the service. So the primary care trust started funding sessional payments, they would say to a practice, if you take on new patients in an afternoon, we'll give you a sessional payment, several hundred pounds, whatever it is. We're not interested in how many UDAs there are, just do it. So they took on new patients, dentists loved it, no UDAs and they could do that within the existing system.

Access centres were set up in areas where there was no NHS dentistry. If there is no NHS dentistry people can be forced into the private sector, I think people should be able to choose to go into the private sector if they want. But they shouldn't go into the private sector because they can't find an NHS dentist. So we set up access centres with salaried people, but it's a very expensive way to deliver care. We gave these areas, where the access centres were, money and said tender for a normal general practice. And that's what they did. Access centres were a tide you over between no access and new practices, practices were more cost effective. One area where we put a lot of extra money in was Hampshire and Dorset. And in one day, I opened five new practices where there had been virtually no NHS dentistry. I remember going back and saying to the minister I'd had my five a day that day, and I'd open five new practices.[111]

Delivering Better Oral Health

We published the first ever guide to evidence-based prevention in primary care, 'Delivering Better Oral Health, an evidence-based toolkit for prevention'.

The person who had the first idea was my deputy, Tony Jenner, because we learned from the PDS pilot that dentists did not know what evidence-based prevention was. Tony said that we ought to produce a guidance document. Sue Gregory, who was president of the British Association for the Study of Community Dentistry, BASCD, became the chair of the working group. The evidence for prevention was all there,

---

[111] For the reception of the 2006 contract see: The introduction of the new dental contract in England – a baseline qualitative assessment Milsom K, Threlfall A, Pine K, Tickle M, Blinkhorn A, Kearney-Mitchell P. British Dental Journal 208 (2008) 59-62. For an assessment of its impact on treatment decisions see: Clinical decision making by dentists, working in the NHS General Dental Services since April 2006. Davies, B., Macfarlane, F. British Dental Journal 209 (2010) E17.

but it was just scattered all around. It was not collated in one document, which is what Delivering Better Oral Health was. So, we said, let's do it. It was published jointly by the Department of Health and BASCD in September 2007.

I'll explain how it happened. Tony got Sue to pull together a working group. And they just collated. I remember Gill Davis[112] used to go round pharmacies looking at toothpaste and reading how much fluoride was in each toothpaste. It was a phenomenal amount of work that went in. She produced a list of toothpastes with the level of fluoride in each one, and sort of rated them.

But at the time, it was all about access. I couldn't get the civil servants interested in this document about prevention, because access was the be all and end all of everything. So, I had a meeting with Rosie Winterton, who was the minister. Rosie was very interested and at the end of any meeting, she always used to ask if there anything else going on that she should be aware of? So I told her that Tony and I were working on this evidence-based prevention document. I explained the background and she said it was interesting and how could she help? So I said, 'well, you could actually help if you drop me an email, and say, 'Thank you for the discussion around an evidence-based toolkit for prevention. I'd like to be kept informed of progress, and I'd like to launch it when it's ready." And I asked her to copy in our Head of Policy, and our Head of Finance in the dental bit of the Department of Health. And could she send that tomorrow morning.

I was in the office and the email came in from the minister's office, and you always open emails from ministers' offices. My office doors were always open, and within about two minutes, I had the Head of Policy and the Head of Finance in my office with steam coming out their ears, saying, 'What are you doing getting the Minister to agree to something which we haven't got funding for?' And they were absolutely livid.

Eventually the Head of Policy said 'you knew exactly what you were doing, didn't you?' If I'd asked him, he would have said no, so the best thing to do was to get it approved, and then tell him it was going to be done. The dental division had a budget of about three and a half billion pounds. The cost for production of the first edition was about 380,000 pounds. So when you're doing end of year reconciliation, 380,000 pounds would get lost in the rounding.

---

[112] Senior Dental officer, Manchester PCT who sat on the working group.

And that had a massive impact. Up until then, toothpaste for the very young contained 440 parts per million of fluoride. and the evidence quite clearly shows that 440 parts per million is not effective in reducing caries. When we published Delivering Better Oral Health, we said that toothpaste for the very young should contain a minimum of 1000 parts per million fluoride compared to 1500, or 1400 parts per million for older people. And within six months, all the major toothpaste manufacturers in the country had changed the concentration of fluoride in toothpaste, and within a further six months, almost all the toothpaste companies around the world had changed the formulation as well.

Fissure sealants were used in the community dental services, but under item-of-service, they were not in the scale of fees and nobody was using fluoride varnish. It was very evidence based, fissure sealants should be used where there was a risk and fluoride varnish for everybody. In the year before we published Delivering Better Oral Health, there was no fluoride varnish used in general practice. The year after there were 5 million which was a mega change in behaviour.

New dental schools

We published a workforce review which showed that we needed more workforce. Actually we needed a more diverse workforce, but we didn't have the broadened scope of practice for dental care professionals at the time. So we got money and opened two new dental schools; I think they were first new dental schools for a long time.

We had a joint implementation group. And we asked for bids, and a lot of people bid for new places in the existing dental schools and quite a few other places bid for new schools.

We wanted them to be graduate entry because that made a shorter course and we would get an outcome quicker. But also, we felt that it brought more mature students into the undergraduate training programme. I'm not a great believer in somebody who's got straight A's making the best dentist or doctor; I think you need a bit of life experience.

One new school was based in Plymouth, but really on the whole southwest peninsula, and the other was based in Preston, UCLAN, the University of Central Lancashire. These were fundamentally different, because there were no dental hospitals. All the teaching was done in outreach in clinics based in the community. There were clinics in Truro, Devonport and Exeter. And in UCLAN they were in Accrington, Carlisle and in Blackpool.

We were told quite clearly by the Dental Schools Council that this was doomed to failure, because you couldn't teach dentistry in the primary care environment, being somebody who had worked for years in primary care I took great exception to that. The Dental Schools Council told us vehemently that this was not going to work. The irony now is that all the old existing dental schools now do a lot of outreach teaching, which is brilliant because the students get far more experience of a more diverse workload in primary care.

But that was quite a challenging time. I think we put in 70 million pounds of capital, some of which went to the existing dental schools to modernise themselves and some of which funded the new building at Plymouth and UCLAN. There was a lot of local impetus to build them. The NHS was very keen to get more dentists in the south-west. The evidence is that if you train people in an area, they stay in that area. Some won't, but a lot will.

I'm still very proud of them. And the government has now said that they want to increase the number of dental places. And because people are so used to outreach teaching, it's going to be much easier this time.

During the period I was Chief Dental Officer we worked very closely with the GDC. If you expand the roles, you've also got to expand the education. And we opened the first dedicated school for dental therapists in Portsmouth, which, again, was based in the community with great support from the NHS in Portsmouth. That's been a great success, and now you've got more schools of therapy around the country. The problem is that the funding for dental therapists doesn't compare to the funding the university gets for training dental students. So that anomaly needs to be addressed. The NHS locally was very keen to fund it and the University of Portsmouth was very keen.

Expanding role of dental care professionals.

Dentistry has moved from a system, when I graduated, where there was a dentist and a dental nurse. In fact, lots of dentists didn't use a dental nurse at the time when I graduated. That's all changed now; there is a huge diversity within the workforce.

If some 70% of the children are free of dental caries, as they are, a well-trained hygienist and therapist can do a risk assessment, and quite happily monitor people where there's no intervention needed or do simple interventions. Why take somebody who is extensively trained and give them work which is very simple?

So we need to make more use of the diversity of the workforce; that is especially true as oral health has much improved. And patients' expectations of their oral health and appearance has changed a lot. We need to grow the diversity of the workforce so that people are working at the top of their skill set. Now we've got extended duty dental nurses, health promoters, hygienists and therapists, and they're all registered with the GDC and they have to work within their scope of practice. They've got the same quality requirements as dentists and that is one of the ways the future of healthcare is going to be delivered, not just in dentistry, but in general health care as well.

The GDC obviously, sets scope of practice but its structure has changed. When I first joined the Department of Health, the Chief Dental Officers of England, Wales, Scotland, and Northern Ireland were all associate members, which meant we attended GDC meetings, took part in debates, but we didn't have voting rights. I was there when they were initially discussing the scope of practice of Dental Care Professionals. There was a working party which looked at scope of practice and came up with a load of recommendations, which were all very sensible. But when it was discussed in Council, the dental members, who used to dominate the council, just added 'under the direction of a dentist' to the end of every chapter. That was not evidence based; it was just pure protectionism.

Sadly, vested interest has had a lot of impact across the board. People who are happy with the situation as is, will oppose change. I remember Eric Rooney once said that change is a constant happening all the time, and if you're fighting to maintain the status quo, you're actually fighting to go backwards. You need to respond to change constantly. And change is a challenge, people don't realise they're better off until change has happened. Remember, people opposed the compulsory wearing of seatbelts vehemently. But who on earth would go back to a situation where we didn't wear seatbelts now?

20. Ron Broadway

Ron Broadway was a regional consultant in orthodontics in Wessex. He described how the orthodontic consultant service started, the early work and organisation and his involvement in education, politics and forensics. He was interviewed by Austin Banner with Sophie Riches in 2019.

******

Bournemouth was the first regional orthodontic consultancy. As in many voluntary hospitals in the country at that time, there were a number of dentists who ran a dental department to treat the deserving poor. When the health service came in some of the people who were more specialised were appointed as consultants. In Bournemouth there was a man called Bobby Torrens who was very much 'go ahead' and they ran a good service in Bournemouth and, as far as I know, he was made a consultant dentist. In balance perhaps he was an oral surgeon but he was appointed as a consultant dentist.

Then they had a committee meeting and decided that they wanted was an orthodontist. So, they went through their management committee up to the Regional Management Hospital Board and it was approved. They advertised the post and John Hooper was appointed just after the NHS had been established. He joined the Royal Victoria Hospital, Bournemouth in 1950.

Voluntary hospitals.

Before the NHS there were two types of hospital. There were the ones run by the county council and the others were voluntary hospitals entirely funded by voluntary funds. The surgeons and physicians who worked there were known as honoraries, they gave up their time for free to work in the hospitals. Some gave up to three days in order to do clinics, operate and see follow ups. This was not entirely altruistic, particularly in the large teaching hospitals, as the students, when qualified, would send their wealthier patients to the honoraries' private practices. All the big London hospitals were voluntary hospitals.

Appointment as a hospital orthodontist

I started as a consultant at the Royal Hampshire County Hospital, Winchester, in May 1960. At my appointment committee John Revens, the Regional Medical Officer, told me that they were going to put me into temporary accommodation, but I wasn't to worry because there was going to be a new hospital within five years. I was naive enough to believe that! That building was there until about four years ago.[113]

As far as I was concerned it was a very good prefabricated building which they hoisted onto the site with a crane. I was asked to design the inside of it. I had three months before I could take up my appointment to work out my contract at the Eastman where I was a senior registrar. I spent time trying to find things out from there, coming down to the region to see the architects and design the department, and, for the time, we had a pretty good department.

My design was based on what we had at the Eastman, I think the modules were 12-foot square, which for a surgery was quite good. They asked what staff I would require; Wessex was pretty good at that. It was all a blank sheet. I had a secretary, a dental nurse and a technician and that was it. A second technician was appointed later when the work increased. The secretary was full-time, she did all the secretarial work for the clinics, I used a reel-to-reel dictation machine. Initially I had one full-time dental nurse and later two part time qualified dental nurses were appointed. They took and processed X-ray films including OPGs and lateral skulls.

My contract was for Winchester, Southampton, Basingstoke and Alton and any other venue that they decided they'd like me to do. I was told that Southampton had been asked if they would like a consultant in orthodontics and the Chief Dental Officer in Southampton, the Community Dental Officer, declined because he said that they couldn't even cope with the amount of decay. But Chadwick, who was the Chief Dental Officer in Winchester, accepted so they got a consultant orthodontist in Winchester.

Winchester is really only a small city, only about 30,000 population. When I started the job, I became a member of the medical staff. There was a Medical Staff Committee which all consultants could attend. I spent a lot of time in medical committees saying, 'And dentistry'. I was certainly accepted by them and served on the local Merit Award

---

[113] He was talking in 2019.

Committee. But none of the medical staff knew what an orthodontist was or did. This was fine from my point of view because I could ask for things, and they didn't know what they were and so they thought they'd better give them to me. That was good.

When I started, I thought, rather naively, that I would be giving advice to general dental practitioners and community dental officers. In the 1960s very few GDPs or community dental officers asked for advice; they wanted me to take on their patients for treatment. But for very straightforward cases I would give detailed advice regarding extractions, design of removable appliances and offers to review their treatment.

I gave talks to BDA sections and I sent out flyers to all the GDPs in the local community saying that I was here and that I would be happy to see their patients and it would be helpful if they could send their study models and any relevant x-rays. But the general standard of study models was very poor, and some of the x-rays were unreadable and I often had to repeat them. Initially, I didn't have panoramic X-rays but we had a cephalostat and it was made by the Saunders-Roe Aircraft Company. A chap came over from Saunders-Roe to see what we wanted, designed it and they made it.

We were next door to the X-ray department, and we used to give the patient the cassette to take round to them and they would develop it and bring it back. I only had one difficulty, a very snooty Winchester lady complained that she was expected to do this. So I told her that the alternative was for me to sign a form for her to go round to X-ray to have it taken and they would probably tell her to come back in a week's time after the films had been reported by the consultant radiologist so she would need another appointment; and her child would have lost three or four days schooling. So she took it.

I gave very detailed advice on the design of the appliances because it was nearly all removable appliances for GDPs. I would design the appliance and told them: Adams cribs and springs and the diameters of the wires and so on, in great detail, and then ask them if they wanted me to review the case, which I would be pleased to do. I can't remember the proportion, but of the ones that I did see again I was sometimes horrified by the appliances and I don't know how the children managed to wear them.

The dentists I was advising had only undergraduate training if they had any at all. So, then the next thing was to run courses for them. Somebody came down from London, the British Postgraduate Medical

Federation. He was Dean of one of the dental schools and he asked if I would I be willing to run some courses for them. That was the beginning of Section 63 courses.

We would bring GDPs into the unit, one half day a week for 6 weeks with one chair. I concentrated on getting them to be able to get decent appliances made. Practical, technical skill rather than clinical skill. Later I also involved the technicians; a lot of the dentists in those days had their own technicians. We had a lab on site as well as X-ray room, office, waiting room and surgery.

I treated a whole range of cases myself. Even as much as pushing an incisor over the bite, even as much as saying 'Get a spatula and bite on that.' An awful lot of treatment was done, referrals escalated fantastically. I think at the peak I was seeing 1000 new patients a year, for everything, advice and treatment.

I did the notes on the same system that we used at the Eastman. When a new patient came in and I'd got all the details, models and X-rays and so on and I'd made a diagnosis and treatment plan, that went into the hospital notes. But we also had our departmental notes because in those days to get hold of the hospital notes every month was a task that the secretary would find extremely difficult.

I went to do clinics at Basingstoke and Southampton. There was no surgery in Southampton General Hospital. They offered me an ex-army wooden chair with an attached spittoon, which they would wheel into an ordinary clinic room in general outpatients, which also served as accident and emergency. Later they found me a surgery in the Western Hospital, on the outskirts of Southampton. There I had a proper dental surgery; I used to take a nurse with me.

I was using removable appliances, Andresen appliances and fixed appliances. They would have been the Eastman type fixed appliances, multi-band, and we had to make our own bands and pull up each band separately. This was before we had pre-formed bands, we had a press to press out brackets which had to be welded onto the band. That was ripple brackets. We'd have to bend up all our own arch wires in various gauges of wire.

I spent most of my time treating rather than giving advice but, when I went to Basingstoke and Southampton, I did more advice than treatment. All the fixed appliance therapy had to be done in Winchester.

Education and training

The advent of the clinical assistant was originally to train general medical and general dental practitioners in a speciality for a limited period of time, so they could go out with their expertise and then they could be replaced by another general practitioner. I did this very strictly and supervised. I think they were paid, but not very much. I varied them: one year a general dental practitioner, the next year would be a community dental officer. They would be with me for a year for one session a week.

By then we had two chairs, the clinical assistant treated selected cases and they were properly supervised. I was treating some patients at the same time, but I didn't have as many patients. We had two chairs in my second department, but there was not a division between them, just a barrier really. And I could hear what they were saying if they were in any difficulty. The nurses were also very good. They could signal you if they didn't think things were going right or something and you'd wander across and say, 'Oh yes, let's have a look' and so on. But it was mainly getting them used to working with removable appliances and then simple fixed appliances. And as time went by with preformed bands and things, they could develop themselves. Although they did get to use fixed appliances within the unit, I doubt whether they did it in their practices because everything is money and it's an investment to start setting yourself up in a practice with all the orthodontic bands and arches and so on. So I doubt whether many of them did it.

The department moved three times, firstly to the former maternity outpatient department, then to the former postgraduate library. At each move we upgraded nearly all the equipment including the waiting room. Then I had a registrar, a nice young man and he stayed for two years, full time with me. He didn't come with me to out-clinics; he was given responsibility to work on his own because that's what the doctors do. He was given new patients to examine and set up a treatment plan. Then we had a session whereby he would present the patients to me with his treatment plan and I would agree or disagree, and we would come to a definitive treatment plan and he would undertake treatment calling for advice as needed.

Later the registrar went to clinics at the new hospital in Basingstoke when Ray Reed was appointed. That worked well. Then I went one step further than that. I went to talk with Clifford Ballard[114] and we came to

---

[114] Professor of Orthodontics at the Eastman. He was the first UK professor of orthodontics, for more about Professor Ballard see Chapter 13.

an agreement whereby one of his registrars would spend their second year in Winchester. They were pretty competent and would have held the Diploma, the D. Orth and an FDS, mostly, by then. There were some very good chaps, a great lot, and they seemed to like spending a year with me. Some would have then gone on to do a senior registrar job somewhere else and others would go into practice.

Vocational Training and Postgraduate Dean

When the new hospital and medical school at Southampton were opened, a Postgraduate Dean was appointed. That was Pat Shackleton and he and John Revens the Regional Medical Officer came and asked if I would like to be the Postgraduate Advisor, as I was going some education. I agreed and they told me to take two or three sessions off to do that. There was no formal appointment, I was just told to take two or three sessions.

Then I started running vocational training, not in orthodontics, in dentistry. I was on the Postgraduate Medical Advisory Committee, the dental section, and various committees. When it came to vocational training, we appointed a GP advisor. It had to be a GP advisor as well as the Dean and we went round inspecting practices who had asked to be training practices. Richard Gorham, the GP advisor, was a strict chap, I was perhaps a bit more laid back about it, but he really made sure they were really up to the mark. We had no lack of trainees wanting to join a practice. The difficulty came at the end of their vocational training year; if there was any vacancy within the practice, they usually filled it. I can't remember how many practices we had but we covered the whole of Hampshire, Wiltshire and Dorset, a big patch.

I started a voluntary vocational training scheme originally. I hoped for a two-year scheme; six months in the hospital service, 6 months in the community service and a year in selected general practice. But I was unable to get funding for the hospital and community posts so the scheme was limited to general practice. A GDP advisor was appointed and applications were sought from GDPs to apply to become trainers.

The University decided that they would promote me to Postgraduate Dental Dean. I was a member of the Conference of Postgraduate Deans and Advisors. I was the first Postgraduate Dental Dean in Southampton. That no longer exists of course because it's now based in Oxford. But Ray Reed followed me as Postgraduate Dental Dean in Southampton, but he was the last. I was the first and he was the last.

The Deanery covered Hampshire, Wiltshire and Dorset. There was quite a lot of work involved. I first worked at the Regional Hospital Board and then at the Postgraduate Centre in Southampton. I was provided with a secretary. The training was directed more towards the general dental practitioner rather than the registrars or specialist practitioner. The registrars were trained by the local consultants. There weren't many of us.

Initially, of course, the BDA was the only source of education. They asked you to give talks. They were always about 7 o'clock in the evening in a pub, they were very well attended. I think initially I went too much into the theoretical Ballardian orthodontics[115].

Management

We managed our own department. The number of times a manager actually came into my department in the whole of the time I was there, without me inviting him or her, could be 10, maybe 20 times. We used to have a little get together with the nurses and technicians and decide whether there was anything we had to do or alter and then we'd go to management and say what we wanted to do.

When we first came to Winchester the management of the hospital used to consist of the hospital secretary, the hospital finance officer, the hospital engineer and I think that was about it. The hospital secretary had a sidekick, a junior and a secretary. If a nurse or secretary wanted to move on or get married, something like that, I would just phone up Miss Street in Mr Perkins' office they would advertise for a replacement. End of story.

As for finance, the routine day to day things you just ordered; obviously there was a budget for that. It was a yearly budget and at the end of the year if you hadn't spent your budget then that money wouldn't be held for you for the next year. You had to spend it or lose it. That was a terrible system because it encouraged people around February or March to spend money completely unnecessarily to use up their budget. I think we got funds through applications to the Medical Staff Committee who had a representative on the Hospital Management Committee. I never had any problem.

---

[115] See: The Ballards and the NHS Professor Clifford Ballard (1910 - 1997) and Orthodontics in the NHS Sophie Riches and Austin J Banner Dental Historian 2019 64 (2) 73-81.

Outside of dentistry I was a member of the Medical Staff Committee and I was a consultant member of the Management Committee for a number of years. My attitude right from the word go was they don't know who you are, they don't know what you do, get involved as much as possible. Try and make yourself indispensable if possible as that's the way to progress and get the system going properly.

I remember an ENT surgeon saying to me 'Don't think because you're not a doctor, you're not important to us.'

Surgery

I did some of my own dental-alveolar surgery when I was first a consultant, such as if there was a canine that needed uncovering; I would have an operating session on a Saturday morning and uncover a canine or take out some supernumeraries. That all stopped very quickly. When I first came, we had an oral surgery clinic once a month staffed from Odstock, Salisbury. When Southampton hospital was built we had a proper surgical department, and then a weekly oral surgeon, in my third department. All of which were prefabricated buildings.

The orthognathic surgery was all done either at Odstock, at the plastic unit, or I think they might have done some at Southampton. If it was done in Southampton Ian Davidson would do the orthodontics there. The oral surgery at Winchester was dentoalveolar surgery.

Research and audit

All the way along we kept records of how many patients we saw, and I think we might even have kept records of the numbers of fixed appliances compared with removable appliances. But the pressure was to get the patients through, get them treated either by the practitioners or by myself and my staff. There wasn't anything much in the way of research. There was the odd paper given by registrars, of course, and I may have done one or two. I was President of the BSSO[116] in 1981 and I had to do something for that. I was a member of the COG[117] Committee and Hon. Sec. for a number of years. I have a feeling that COG was formed as we were concerned that we were in danger of losing parity with oral surgery.

When we had finished treatment and discharged the patient after review, our notes were put in the hospital notes and kept for as long as

---

[116] British Society for the Study of Orthodontics, British Orthodontic Society.
[117] Consultant Orthodontic Group.

hospital notes are kept. I doubt if anybody ever went back to look at them retrospectively.

College of Surgeons

I was made a life member of the BDA, which has enabled me to keep an interest in dentistry throughout my retirement. It helps when anyone asks me about dentistry to reply that I retired in 1992 and things have moved on since then.

I was elected in about 1980 to the Faculty of Dental Surgery RCS, and served for eight years, becoming Chairman of the Education Committee for some time. This involved inspecting the orthodontic departments of some dental schools for recognition of their departments by the College. It was usually just two of us from the College. Usually it was Jack Tulley and I, we did a lot of it.

I spent 32 happy years in Winchester and by the contract of the day had to retire on my 65th birthday, though I did stay on for one more year as Postgraduate Dean.

Up to about two years before I retired, I thought orthodontics was going to be going well ahead. That there would be more practitioners practising orthodontics and wanting advice, but one would not be doing as much treatment oneself, except on really difficult cases and cooperating with the oral surgeons. But I think it went downhill a bit after that. One consultant told me I was an old-fashioned consultant because I spent most of my time at the chairside. I said, 'Yes that's what I was paid for.'

Forensic dentistry

I did quite a lot of forensic work. We had a Home Office pathologist on the staff, and he asked if I would help him with any cases involving teeth and dentistry. This work was for Hampshire Constabulary. There were lots of cases, mostly skeletons dug up by construction workers. Mostly Roman and pre-Roman and that sort of thing. They'd bring in a mandible, or something, with very worn teeth and you'd look at it and say 'This is very interesting but it is very old.' If it was not within living memory, it was ok. Then I got involved in dental identification of patients in car accidents, burning and murder cases with bite marks.

I had no formal training in forensics, only what I'd read, and I think orthodontists were really quite well trained for a lot of that because we can assess age from x-rays much better than most other dental people.

I found that being cross examined in the High Court by a barrister is probably more wearing than any oral exam I've ever had. For one of them, I was there for half the morning and for most of the afternoon. The chap kept asking me about the histology. I kept saying that it was outside my expertise; and in the end the judge intervened and said 'He has already told you that he is not an expert in that.'

I didn't do any after I retired; I came off the register because I didn't want to go on anyway. But the first question a defending barrister would ask you is 'How many cases have you had of this and when was the last time you saw this?'

It was very smelly and very gruesome at times. I had a case of three sailors in a car, they were burnt to a cinder. The whole camp had been given a weekend leave and no one knew who they were, and they needed to know. I did find out who they were, by 4 o'clock in the morning. And I got a commendation from the Assistant Chief Constable; it's amazing how you can keep awake when you have to. I had to look at all their dental records, being in the service they had their records. And then, bingo.

21. Dolly Terfus

Dolly was the daughter of a Jewish family who were refugees from Russia and subsequently Germany. She told how her father set up a laboratory in central London which she inherited and described the work of one of the first woman owned dental laboratories. She was interviewed by Stephen Simmons in 2011.

******

Jewish refugees from Russia and then Germany

My parents came over from Europe in 1939. My father was an established technician in Germany, having left Russia when he was 12, at the time of the pogroms, and came to Germany with his sister and his mother. He was a student of technology, originally a fabric designer, but he became a dental technician in Germany.

He fled Germany very late in 1939 and arrived here in England. A lot of European Jewry were offered either to go into the British army and serve or be interned on the Isle of Wight. My father, because he was saved by England, said he would go into the army but he was allowed days off to continue his profession.

He went with the Pioneer Corps, I think it was the 178th Company, or something like that, to the West Country. When he was demobbed we were living in Taunton, which is where my sister was born, and we also lived in Chard. He was then asked by my mother to find a job in London, near a school or a shopping area, and he found a position with a Hungarian technician. Her name was Lakatos and she had a laboratory, number 29 Beaumont Street at the corner of Marylebone High Street. He was a manager there for a year.

Setting up a laboratory in Marylebone

Over that time, he befriended the rector of St Marylebone church, a Reverend Matthews. How they met I don't know, but he was offered a place in Marylebone school, the whole of the upper floor where he was allowed to live with his family and have a laboratory. It was at 63 Marylebone High Street, and the rooms are still there. He set up his laboratory one year after having left the Lakatoses.

Over that time he would have befriended various, what were known as travellers, representatives, and one of the suppliers was a Norman Rayne, who made Rayway motors, and a lot of technicians will know what they were. This is prior to my birth. He was given a present of a Rayway motor, and it lasted for a very long time. I think it was at least 50 years old before it died. Norman Rayne was very kind to my father. I think they collected money to help him set up. Obviously, I don't know all the details because I was really very tiny, but I do know that the Rayway motor was given to him as a present.

He set up his laboratory in the school. And because of his connections with the European dentists, all the dentists he worked for were from Europe. They all spoke German, the suppliers and the technicians. They could all speak English, but there was no need to.

A new innovation - porcelain jacket crowns

My father was one of the very first to undertake a course, which was set up in Weybridge, to learn how to make porcelain jacket crowns. That's what we called them then. This course lasted for, as far as I know, a weekend. I took him there, he finished the course and then, unfortunately, he died. That would have been in the middle to the late 1960s. Porcelain, which was quite an innovation, was coming onto the market, and prior to that he did absolutely everything in the laboratory, whether it was gold work, prosthetics or vulcanite.

Prosthetic technician was not feminine

Having grown up around teeth and because I was good with my hands, not the academic that my sister was, I thought I'd join him, but for three years he said no because it wasn't feminine and that it was hard work being a prosthetic technician. I really begged him and eventually, after three years of nagging, he said right, okay, you will come and you will be apprenticed to me.

It wasn't a career that people knew very much about. It wasn't publicised. It wasn't anything that anybody in school would recommend as a profession because they didn't know about it. Everyone knew of dentists. I worked with my father for about ten years before he died.

That was about 1951 and the apprenticeship was five years long and you stood at the master's elbow. He told you what to do and you then sat down and you did it until you got it right, even if it meant doing the same thing a hundred times. When you got it right, then you proceeded onto the next one.

Dental mechanics

I don't know whether the City & Guilds was around then. I don't know if any colleagues of mine went to do that. It was Borough Polytechnic where you went one day a week to learn dental technology, which is what it became. We were called dental mechanics. Dental technicians didn't come in as a word till a long time afterwards.

When you had finished your apprenticeship, a dentist that you had worked for would then sign you off and would say, 'I have known so and so for this length of time. They have worked for me; their work is acceptable.' And then sign a letter, which was then presented to the Joint Council for the Craft of Dental Technicians, and you applied for registration with the letter. They would then send back confirmation, saying you were now a qualified dental technician, or dental mechanic. They had never met you or saw anything you produced, only knowing you by name and by reputation. There was no paperwork required, but the profession was very small, especially here in the West End. There weren't that many laboratories and everybody knew one another, so the registration board would no doubt have heard of you.

My certificate, because a woman had never applied before, has got 'he' and I then went and put an 's' in front of it so it was 'she'. I've still got that today. And after my father died, to the best of my knowledge I was amongst the first female technicians to have her own laboratory and to be totally self-employed, but I elected to stay on my own because of the aggravation that my father suffered with employing anybody.

No rules and regulations

There were no rules and regulations. We were a very new body of people. Registration was unheard of. You just set up and, provided you had the clientele, you could go anywhere, do anything. Nothing was vetted, there was no overseer. But this Joint Council was really very new. I think they wanted to formalise it.

There was a long distance between that and the Medical Devices Directive, which was a form of Kite Mark. It was actually to register the laboratories, so that you had a professional Kite Mark, but it didn't prove that you were any good at your profession. Then you became like a collective body of people.

The Dental Care Professional Register

In about 2008 the General Dental Council decided they were going to make a Dental Care Professional Register, to which every single technician had to apply. But because I am the age I am, I came in what was known as the 'grandfather clause', which means you had no paper documents. It was only what you could do, no paper was required. You had a letter in the middle of the year, provided you applied for registration by December. It would only cost £94 after December. There was a questionnaire, and all I filled in was 'grandfather clause' with my age, whereupon they then sent me a piece of paper and it says, 'Dental Technician, verified experience in dental technology' and that was all that was required. This was to be updated annually, and I retired in 2010, so I only had the next year after that, where the registration fee had gone up. What you got was the permission to practise as a technician but, once again, nobody came to judge the quality of work.

Vulcanite, nylon and acrylic

Going back to the birth of technology, dentures were made of vulcanite, which was a form of rubber, for which you had to have special equipment which was liable to explode, depending on how good the equipment was. But the dentures were brown or a deep rusty red. They were only one colour and the teeth were made of porcelain with gold pins in the back which were then secured into the vulcanite. The system of processing dentures has never changed. It's the lost wax system.

After vulcanite you then came onto acrylic, which is a plastic. They did, at one stage, try nylon to see whether dentures couldn't break, but nylon did break. We used nylon in the laboratory and I remember one of our dentists was experimenting in front of a patient trying to sell him this nylon, and of course it broke. But he quickly recovered himself and said, 'Oh this isn't a nylon denture.' But you couldn't repair it. So nylon then was discarded and we still use acrylic but in different forms. Vulcanite has vanished.

Casting gold

My father's gold casting equipment is in a museum in Kent. It was a very old-fashioned method of casting gold. It was a really small furnace. It was a rotund tube that sat on four legs, and it had a little funnel. There was a small cradle which was in the middle of it and you opened up the top, as if you were opening up a lid. The cradle inside held a small cylinder in which whatever you were casting, whether it was a tooth, a bridge or something else, was inserted into a special plaster. You waited until the furnace had heated up the flask and you could see the top would go red. It was then put onto another contraption, which was the casting machine. The gold was then forced into the small cylinder, and all this was done by hand. I don't think the centrifugal system had even been invented then.

The casting was whirled around. There was a small pot at the end of a chain and that was controlled by a small wooden handle and you then, literally, swung it around the room.

If you lost control over the swing and the little pot at the end became loose or limp, the gold vanished into the walls and that was it, so you started all over again.

I would hate to tell you how much gold is embedded in the walls of the laboratory, which I don't think I'll ever find. It was an art, and you practised until you got it right. The first time I did it, I was absolutely petrified. I thought this thing is going to go all around the room, which of course it did.

That was all before natural gas came in. To heat this up, you had a gun. It looked like a little gun, which was controlled with gas and air. It had long tubes connected to bellows. If you can imagine bellows on legs, which is what it was. It stood on legs with a foot control, with which you pumped the air from the bellows into the little gun. You controlled it with a lever so that the flame was fierce enough to melt the gold. Now all this, of course, has been superseded by the centrifugal force, but that is how you did it then. I held onto the equipment because it was so ancient and it's now in a museum in Kent. I didn't want to throw it away because this is our history of how technology evolved.

The master or the owner of the laboratory then would be quite competent in working in gold and if he was doing prosthetics, he would do both. He would do the gold work for bridges, or even gold dentures, depending on if somebody was wealthy enough and wanted a gold denture. Chrome was sent out to specific laboratories who specialised in chrome dentures but, prior to that, it was stainless steel.

Stainless steel was a lot heavier but there are people who are allergic to the components of chrome dentures and stainless steel was ideal for them. There are also people who are allergic to the monomer in acrylic dentures. It can cause blistering and they then would have stainless or gold.

The older technician was accomplished in doing the whole thing, right across the board. When the field became wider, he or she found they couldn't do the whole range, so then you elected either to become a prosthetic technician or a ceramist.

Prior to light-cure machines, to make a specific denture, you would have to make special trays and they were made of shellac, brown, green, pink, and if you got that on your fingers, you had the almightiest burn. But then that was superseded by light-cured trays, for which you had a little light-cure machine. It was much cleaner and easier; you could do three or four at a time.

Asbestos

We didn't know about asbestosis in those days and I had a colleague that actually died of asbestosis. There was a lot of asbestos used then because the furnace would have to sit on an asbestos table and so the heat from the furnace didn't go into the ceiling of the room, there was an asbestos cover, it was white asbestos. The small cylinders in which the gold was cast were lined with asbestos strips, which you got in a little box from the suppliers and our suppliers were Claudius Ash, L Porrow or Cottrell. We had no idea, then, about the damage that would cause to the lungs.

Articulators and new equipment

All we ever had were straight line articulators. Now there are those big three-dimensional articulators. We didn't use face bows. Now they have mixers for mixing plaster, we just used a spatula. Now it's done electronically. This is another thing; you've got computers which do all the milling and all of that. Computers are involved in a big way. We didn't have computers.

Getting and keeping clientele

To acquire clientele, your reputation very often preceded you and dentists might ring you up and say, I hear you work for so and so, would you work for me? They would either come to you or you would present yourself to them, talk about it, taking with you your worksheets and your price list. For private work there are no rules at all on what you charge. Pre 1948,[118] you charged whatever you thought was right. The dentist didn't tell you what he charged, but you sort of found out amongst your colleagues and you worked around that. After 1948, when the guidelines came in and the dentist was then told how much he could charge, you'd have to drop your price or you were then limited, within a range of figures. Occasionally things went wrong so you were then out of pocket.

---

[118] The National Health Service was introduced in 1948.

When I first started working, in the late 1950s, you would charge maybe 12, 13 pounds for a full denture, which then was a lot of money. It was all relative. But nowadays you're talking thousands. I don't think I ever charged thousands, but I was charging in the hundreds. The payment system was, that at the end of each calendar month, a statement was presented to the dentist, who, if they were good, would pay you with a cheque within two or three days. Some used the whole calendar month. There were others who decided that they would wait a little longer and I know colleagues who have waited for much longer than that. And we can be talking about thousands of pounds. They will be paid, probably, immediately by their patients, but the poor old technician didn't get paid until a lot later and we would very often suffer a cash flow problem. Chasing dentists for money has always been a bugbear with every single technician, and that hasn't altered from the 1950s until the present day.

Working hours and conditions

The working hours were bizarre. You worked until the job was complete, which meant very often if your shelf was full of work, you got up at the crack of dawn and you worked until you were finished, and if that meant working until 11, 12 at night, you did. I remember, often, coming into work and finding my father had worked the night through and was still at the polishing lathe.

My working day originally started about seven o'clock in the morning but when I got really busy and I knew I had a lot on, I would get up at 5:30 and be at my bench at seven and I stayed there until I was finished. I did my own errands because I thought it was important to stay in contact with the dentist, and that was something that my father had told me. He said, 'Always talk to your dentist because that way, they understand you and you understand what they want.' You worked weekends, no time off. I didn't go on a holiday for almost 20 years. You were always at the bench.

There were no masks. I wore gloves because my ex-mother-in-law had told me, always to look after your hands. She was the very first female anaesthetist in London. I always wore gloves for polishing, mixing plaster, investing, boiling out, everything, but obviously not for finishing dentures. Masks, no. They were around and when the Medical Devices Directive came out, we were supposed to wear them, but you'll find we didn't. They do now. I didn't have ventilation in the laboratory, I had an open window. It worked, there were no extractors.

22. Philip Sutcliffe

Phillip was inspired towards children's dentistry and epidemiology research. He became an academic in Edinburgh and later Dean and had to oversee the closure of the Edinburgh undergraduate dental school. He spoke to Mark McCutcheon in 2012.

*****

I was born in Todmorden in the West Riding of Yorkshire on the 17th May 1935. Until about 1950, my father was a foreman working in a cotton mill in Rochdale in Lancashire. My mother used to be a weaver in Todmorden. She didn't work after they got married, so she was a housewife as long as I knew her. I guess they both left school at 14, something like that.

I was the first person in the family to go to university, undoubtedly because of the freedoms brought about by the Education Act of 1944, which opened up the grammar schools. And my parents leant on me until I got to university. I think I was pretty awful academically, but I got good O-Levels and that was the first sign that there was something happening. I did maths, physics and chemistry A-levels and I got a place to do physics at Leeds University.

Why dentistry?

At that time I was wondering about the idea of physics as a career. It seemed to me that I would be either teaching or doing research, and neither seemed very appealing. So I went to the library, and I saw something about dentistry and I knew those subjects would get me into a dental school.

I thought the chap who treated me in the School Dental Service, when I was about ten, was pretty awful, and I thought I could probably do better than him. So I wrote to the Dean of Science, and asked if I could change to dentistry. He wrote back, and he said that the Professor of Dentistry would be pleased to accept me. So I went to the dental school on the 4th of October 1954.' I was not interviewed, I just turned up on the first day.

Dentistry was an unpopular subject in those days. Dentists had a bad reputation as money grubbers. The popular belief was they earned stupendous amounts of money providing patients mainly with dentures, at the beginning of the Health Service.

Leeds University

On 4th of October 1954, I was among 40 students who started at Leeds Dental School. Half the year came from Norway. They had only one dental school in Oslo in those days; we took several Norwegians in every year.

My first year was extremely confusing. I did botany and zoology because I'd never done that ever before, and physics and chemistry of dental materials. I enjoyed botany and zoology but I was completely confused by the physics and chemistry of dental materials. We did things on gold, plaster, porcelain, amalgam. I had no idea what they were or what I was going to do with them. At the same time, the chinks were filled in with dental mechanics, which went on for two years.

I never met a graduate dentist in those first two years apart from one and his name was Mr Thornton and he ran the lab and was a Bachelor of Dental Surgery. He spent some time with me because I simply could not wax up full upper and lower dentures properly. He showed me how to just spin it through the flame of a Bunsen burner 18 inches high, and that was a great revelation. But I can still remember Mr Hughes, my instructor, a very nice guy, but I had great difficulty in understanding what he was teaching me.

The beginning of dentistry wasn't great for me. I failed the pathology exam, but I slowly woke up so that by the time I got to the resit I had settled down with a new textbook. That experience taught me how to read and how to learn; from then on, things got a lot better.

From dental mechanics you progressed to working in the prosthetic clinic, mainly on full upper and lower impressions. For the degree examination at the end of two years, you made special trays for your patient and then took impressions. The examiner then was Professor Hutchinson from Edinburgh University. He must have tolerated what I produced, so I got through that exam.

We went through the phantom head laboratory, working on extracted teeth which were mounted. I have little of a memory of it, but, as we progressed through, I can remember my teachers very well, certainly in restorative dentistry. And then the most inspiring teacher for me was

Douglas Jackson,[119] who taught children's and preventive dentistry. He was an excellent teacher and just as I'd liked and followed my physics teacher as a schoolboy, I did the same with Douglas Jackson. And after I qualified and had been away for a bit, I went back to work in his department as a research fellow in preventive dentistry and then my career really took off. He was just a good teacher, youngish and enthusiastic. I qualified in 1959.

Paediatric dentistry in the USA

Just before I qualified I applied to North Western University in Chicago for a residency in children's dentistry at a paediatric dental hospital there. That gave me teaching in paediatric dentistry from North Western University and clinical practice in the Children's Memorial Hospital. I did that for a year.

It was at the very end of the fashion of going to the States. North Western was popular because it had always welcomed students from abroad. It was the school where Black had been Dean, many years before, so the whole idea of classification of cavities was born in that school. [120] Several people that I've come across since spent some time at North Western. Being with postgraduate students and post-doc students from other disciplines and other universities just seemed a very attractive life. It's amusing that I didn't do physics to avoid teaching and research and I walked into academic life to do teaching and research.

North Western was one of the schools which attracted Geoffrey Slack who became Dean of the London Dental Hospital and another big figure in my time in preventive and children's dentistry.[121] He began his serious academic life in Liverpool and spent some time at North Western. I thought they taught to a higher standard and were more demanding than I had experienced at Leeds. I thought I was better placed in an understanding of the basic clinical sciences, more pathology, bacteriology and more medicine and surgery. They were much better at restoring teeth than I was. That's something I had to learn.

North America kicked me off. When I came back I hadn't a job, I worked maximum part-time in the School Dental Service in Rochdale where was I brought up. I worked in the surgery next door to the school

---

[119] Douglas Jackson see chapter 23.
[120] Dr GV Black, 1836-1915, who devised the still used classification of dental cavities.
[121] Geoffrey Slack see also chapters 23, 24. Also: Geoffrey Layton Slack OBE (Mil), CBE, TD, BDS, DDS, FDSRCS, FDS Glas, FFDRCSi Dip Bact (1912-1991). Gelbier S. Journal of Medical Biography. 2014 Feb 22 (1) 19-31.

dentist who I thought had been cruel to me as a child. He didn't recognise me but came in and said what a pleasure it was to have somebody like me working next to him. I nearly died. The dentist in charge of the School Dental Service there gave me two pieces of instruction, 'We don't use rubber dam, it rots,' and 'We don't fill Ds, we take them out.'

School Dental Service

When I was working in the school service the caries experience was very high, which was a matter of great concern. There was a lot of caries in first permanent molars where a lot of the deciduous teeth were carious. When I came back from the States and travelled home, I was so struck by the appalling visual effect of people's teeth on the train, teeth missing, teeth openly carious, wherever you sat. That has completely vanished these days. It was much worse than in north America. That was about 1960.

Eastman Dental Hospital

After about a year a registrar post was advertised at the Eastman Dental Hospital in London and so I went there and saw the Dean who had been the Dean at Newcastle Dental School,[122] and I explained my career and said I was interested in their registrar post in children's dentistry. He gave me a piece of paper and a pencil and he said, 'Take this down.' And he then dictated a model letter of application, 'Dear Sir, I wish to apply for the post of... the following gentlemen have agreed to act as referees. I will be happy to attend for interview should you call me. Yours faithfully.... I sent in that letter and I was called for an interview and I was appointed registrar in paediatric dentistry under a man called Dick Stevens.

While working in the School Dental Service, I'd kept in touch with the Leeds dental school. I had been to see Douglas Jackson and explained what I was up to. I can't remember anything specifically he said, but he must have nudged me in the right direction and saw I wanted some sort of post in paediatric dentistry that would take me up the ladder.

Inventions at the Eastman

It was very enjoyable. Dick Stevens was an amazing man. He was an inventor, really. He'd worked a lot in the development of air rotors. Air rotors just came in while I was at North Western and the paediatric dentists who were teaching me, one in particular, a very distinguished

---

[122] Professor Robert Bradlaw.

man, said there was no place for an air rotor in children's dentistry, far too dangerous, far too fast, unacceptable to children.

So, at the Eastman I met Dick Stevens, who'd done a lot of basic work on air rotors. He came to a halt when he realised that the burr we needed would need to be of a smaller diameter than the conventional burr and he didn't think manufacturers would make a change of that order. And then the Dean at the Eastman suggested he should try something else so he invented a rotating mirror, a hand mirror for the mouth which spun around so that it would throw off the moisture. It was good, but the problem was if it wobbled, the image was poor.

In those days, he was working towards a jet injector. Anaesthetic drugs would be injected into your gum under pressure and it avoided the use of a needle. It worked, but it was a bit hair-raising if you were his registrar because he'd come in, smoking a cigarette, put it down on the instrument tray, and say, 'Philip, I've had another go, do you mind opening your mouth.,' and I'd feel a bit more anaesthetic going into my palate and then he'd go away quite satisfied. He really was a very interesting man. He was a consultant in paediatric dentistry and probably honorary senior lecturer.

Fluoride toothpaste trial

After I'd been at the Eastman for a couple of years, Douglas Jackson, back in Leeds, had secured funding for what was to be described as the demonstration trial for a fluoride dentifrice. Procter & Gamble financed three trials at the London Dental Hospital, Birmingham Dental Hospital and Leeds. And we would do a controlled prospective trial of the value of stannous fluoride toothpaste in 11-year-old children and we'd run this for three years. That would have been 1962/63. They'd been established in the States, and it was accepted there that it reduced caries experience, but Procter & Gamble wanted to introduce it in three dental schools to provide proof that they would work in Britain.

This was a momentous time in the impact of fluoride toothpastes but we didn't realise it at the time. I examined 1,000 children in West Riding grammar schools. We chose grammar schools because we thought they'd be keen. We wanted people who could be relied upon to brush their teeth. The locations were the grammar schools at Batley, Castleford, Morley, Normanton, Otley, Pontefract and Tadcaster.

I think Douglas Jackson was a leading figure, Geoffrey Slack was in London and Peter James was in Birmingham,[123] and together with John Mansbridge in Edinburgh[124] they were the leading people in dental epidemiology at the time and I think that's why the funding went their way.

I was taken on to do the clinical examinations. Every year the children were split up into control and test groups and I examined them in the proper way, they didn't know which group they were in, I didn't know which group they were in, and recorded their caries experience annually for three years. We looked at the results. I had also taken on another group of 500 children who were a different sort of control, who were just left alone in case there was an improving effect, if you like, upon the control group in the clinical trial. So, I was really looking at 1,500 grammar school children annually. We measured the decrease in caries increment; it seemed quite small and I don't think my results differed greatly from those of the other two centres.

We were disappointed by that because we knew from water fluoridation, we could expect something like a 50 percent reduction in caries experience. But I followed on with my 1,000 grammar school children after the trial ended until they all left school at 18. I then chose the control group and so from that I had a continuous study of caries, gingivitis and other conditions in a mouth running from the age of 11 through to 18, and that became the basis of my PhD. I had also written a master's degree under Douglas Jackson's guidance a bit earlier. So, I came away from Leeds in 1971, with an MSc, or a Master of Dental Surgery, and PhD. That was what I got out of it.

Early indicators of caries experience and fissure sealants

This research pointed towards early indicators of a high caries experience. I could see which first permanent molars were likely to be extracted according to their caries experience of the different surfaces and the ones that would survive. But these became completely useless because caries experience in children fell and there wasn't the same need for these indicators of high caries experience for high pressure preventive dentistry.

Dick Stevens was playing with fissure sealants and he liked to ram gold foil into non-carious first permanent molars, held in with an epoxy

---

[123] Peter James also see chapters 12, 23.
[124] Mansbridge see also chapter 23.

resin or something of the sort. People were playing with the idea of fissure sealants. It wasn't unusual in my undergraduate days and graduate days to run black copper cement into the fissures of first permanent molars to prevent them from becoming carious. A lot of the things which we take for granted now were at their beginning and preventive dentistry was working.

I had a lot of fun with gingivitis. I wrote a paper on the relationship between gingivitis and puberty, following on the papers of relationship between gingivitis and pregnancy. Of course, it took longer in puberty. I still don't know whether I got it right, but that attracted the right sort of attention from a distinguished periodontologist in Scandinavia and caused Geoffrey Slack, who I've talked about before, to say, 'Why don't you chuck children's dentistry and come and work in my department in periodontology?' but I was keen on children's dentistry in those days.

Lecturer at Leeds

After a couple of years as research fellow at the Eastman, I moved back to Leeds as a lecturer in children's and preventative dentistry. I was there from about 1962/63 until 1971. The PhD was expected. I didn't do an FDS because Douglas Jackson said he thought it was a waste of time; it was more important to do research. I think he was wrong about that. And Freddy Hopper, who was the Dean at Leeds, really would have preferred me to do a Fellowship, but I didn't.

Research better than Fellowship

I didn't do a Fellowship, but I did the other things. Freddy Hopper was designing a new dental school at Leeds. He saw that I'd finished my PhD, and he made me his sort of gofer and he said he'd like a bit of help in designing that school and would I like to join in on that, and so in my last months at Leeds I picked up the habits of designing and building a dental school; it was a bit of fun.

By 1971, I wanted a new environment and there weren't many jobs. There was a job of senior lecturer/consultant at the London Dental Hospital and I'd done a stint in London and I quite liked it, but I didn't really want to live in London again. And then the job turned up in Edinburgh, so I applied for that. That caused Edinburgh some difficulty because I now realise that although I had a PhD and my future Professor, David Watt, valued that, I hadn't got my Fellowship and that was a real problem for them. After all, the Edinburgh Dental School, their examining body from the very beginning had been the College of Surgeons and it was natural enough to go through either the Higher

Dental Diploma, which was John Mansbridge's qualification in Edinburgh, or through to the FDS which was just beginning. I hadn't got it. But when I was asked why not, I had said, 'Well, you know, the regulations show you can become a consultant by other routes than going through the Fellowship.' That's all I could say. There was a bit of a delay, but I was appointed after a few days. And I came up to Edinburgh.

Edinburgh Senior Lecturer

I started in Edinburgh in November 1971 as the senior lecturer in children's dentistry in David Watt's department, restorative dentistry. The disciplines were prosthodontics, conservative or restorative dentistry, children's dentistry. It was strange to find myself cut off from preventive dentistry. That was run by John Mansbridge, a very distinguished, quiet Professor of Preventive Dentistry at Edinburgh. He had run the demonstration trials of water fluoridation in Ayr and Kilmarnock, and he'd done a lot of meticulous epidemiology in its very early days, a very distinguished man.

Research nursery school children

But preventive dentistry being cut off from me in a way was good and I did more research. I looked at nursery school children. They were rarely examined in those days and I looked at about 1,000 three- and four-year-olds in State nursery schools in Edinburgh when I first came here. I saw that if you were in the nursery school in Morningside your average DMF, decayed, missing and filled teeth, might have been half. If you were in some of the other areas, Craigmillar, the value would be four or five. Those were the social differences which were always obvious at that time.

I think it was seen that there were social differences. They wouldn't have been seen to be the cause but to be associated with bad dental habits, and that shone through even in those very young children. Looking for correlations, as you always do, the best I found in local Edinburgh evidence, was that in areas like Craigmillar they were also remarkable for the higher proportion of households that had their electrical supply cut off because people couldn't pay, and a hypothesis I used to put about, with my tongue rammed firmly in my cheek, was well clearly their decay was up because they couldn't use their electric toothbrushes.

I enjoyed doing that, and I stuck with nursery school children all the time. In those days, it's probably still true, dental students don't belong to extended families and dental students rarely have much experience of very young children. So I used to take them, instead of doing whatever it was I should have been teaching them, into nursery schools. We would go in small groups to nursery schools and the students would talk to the children, join in their play, open their mouths, look at their teeth and talk about teeth. In that way I wanted them to get to know what the mind of a three and a four-year-old was like and how best to approach them. But I enjoyed that and I think the students did.

Teaching vs research

The idea was I'd do six clinical sessions and four non-clinical sessions each week. That was a five-day week, but in fact in those days we had clinics on Saturday mornings, which everybody hated, partly because they were the preferred clinic for busy working parents. The staff was always only half the number because you got alternate Saturdays off. We all breathed a sigh of relief when certain technical graduates within the hospital refused to work on Saturday morning, and so we said thank God for that.

I mentioned earlier that Geoffrey Slack had said, 'Why don't you come and do periodontology with me?' but I didn't want to. He also said, 'Don't go to Edinburgh, the human relationships there are appalling.' People didn't get on. I don't know that they were worse than in any other dental school, but there was a fair amount of disagreement. I wouldn't have said that it was remarkable if you were on the staff. I don't know as to what extent it communicated itself elsewhere.

There was the dental hospital but the academic departments were spread about the neighbourhood around. Orthodontics was far away; it was more or less where the present institute is in Lauriston Place. Dental materials were in a building which no longer exists, across the road from the dental hospital in Chamber Street. I think it was next door to, or had been, a Chinese restaurant. Restorative dentistry was on George IV Bridge; oral medicine became another outlying station further along George IV Bridge towards the High Street. So, there was a lot of walking around. Slowly the academic departments coalesced into High School Yards and that relieved the congestion around the dental hospital itself.

When I came to Edinburgh in 1971 the curriculum was very congested. And my memory is that it was a four-year course, but that would have made it five with the entry of Scottish Highers because their basic sciences needed augmenting. Now gradually, I think four years became five years. So, the congested curriculum at Edinburgh slowly became decongested as regulations came through to extend to a common five-year curriculum.

Appointment of Deans

John Boyes was the Dean when I came, and he persisted until about 1977/78. He was a very quiet man. His line was oral surgery, and he taught, essentially, in the admissions department in the front hall. That was his discipline and his chosen area of teaching. He had been at the dental hospital in Newcastle before he came up, but he was an Edinburgh man. He would have been qualified in medicine and dentistry. When he retired, he was followed by Graham Charlton, in restorative dentistry. And that marked the end of the Deans for life. Until then, people who were appointed the Dean of a Dental School largely stuck with it. Freddy Hopper was Dean for the whole of his career in Leeds. But gradually the fashion for having a dean who was dean for a period became the predominant one.

When Graham Charlton retired, by then the Deans were elected by the staff and so John Southam was elected Dean and he stayed on for several years and then I was elected Dean after him. And John Southam and I went through the form of annual elections so the staff were on our side. Every year you were asked if you wanted to be Dean again or if others wanted to be Dean and you were elected.

I know that electing Deans became something of a problem because when Vice Chancellors became the ones to be held to account for the universities then they responded by saying, 'Well, we must return to a system of either acceptability of Deans or at least the selection of Deans because we can't be accountable for people who are washed up by the populace.' So there was a modification. But that was certainly popular in several dental schools and that's certainly how things developed here at Edinburgh.

In 1978, John Mansbridge retired, and I applied for his Chair in Preventive and Social Dentistry. I was lucky. Within the department was Bruce Hunter, who went on to be a consultant in paediatric dentistry at Cardiff. Lowna Scowick came into the department from Denmark. She was a live wire with a good understanding of communication and the rest of it in preventive dentistry. Andy Blinkhorn, another communicator, went on to Glasgow, I think, then Australia, all sorts of places. So there have been some interesting people.

We started an MSc in Preventive Dentistry. There were certainly Chief Dental Officers in the United Kingdom who were in the department and did our MSc. The course was in collaboration with the Department of Public Health in the Medical School and so they were taught a lot of the basics of prevention and preventive medicine and the approaches and I would see that they had appropriate teaching in dentistry and they would write their dissertation in dentistry, so that's how it developed.

I always enjoyed teaching children's dentistry and preventive dentistry and statistics the way we did it; and we did some innovations. I always enjoyed it. I don't know whether the students did, but we did. The students were good. I'm not just saying that. A former Chief Dental Officer of Scotland and later on in England said that he always thought that Edinburgh was a class act. I think we got a good quality of student.

One difficulty for us in dentistry was that our students came from the whole of the UK and they returned to the UK and were spread and were not at a later point seen as contributing to dental health and manpower in Scotland.

Choosing students and managing children

Dentistry had all changed from when I began; it became a sought-after profession. In my undergraduate days at Leeds, our class of 40 had two girls, one Norwegian and one English. We remember those two girls very well. By now, there are more girls going into dental schools than men. That's one of the great changes. And similarly, people seek to do dentistry; it's highly competitive.

I don't remember when I thought gosh, things are changing. What I remember was that, as I got into the business of interviewing students for admission, you had to be jolly careful that you didn't choose too many, and so it was a fearful balance. And you had to set up your own rules of what you were looking for. What was I looking for? Competence in the subject, yes; an interest in something outside school, yes; an attitude towards caring; I think those were my criteria for choosing a student. And we got some very good people.

There was never enough time for research and in looking back I should have devoted more time to it. But I enjoyed children's dentistry. I thought that there was a time when people didn't understand children and didn't know how to approach them. In the States, for example, if a child was frightened and played up, one approach was to put your hand over the child's mouth and squeeze their nostrils and whisper in his ear, 'Now just calm down and then I'll take my hand away.' And I thought that was excessively cruel.

When I began in children's dentistry, it was usual to separate parents or mothers from the child and to deal with the child alone in the surgery. I thought that was wrong. With very young children, they're connected to their mother and mothers are connected to their children and I thought it was most important to have the mother and the child together in the surgery. Mothers didn't enjoy it, children didn't always, but it was a way of establishing that you could be trusted and that you could get on with this job which required a lot of cooperation, and you were working towards the child coming in by himself.

Douglas Jackson, who I've said was a great influence, was interesting. If things were not going quite the right way, he'd grab a child's head like a rugby ball, so that it's there, he'd get on with the dentistry and then he'd say, 'Come on, give me a kiss.' And I've seen him roll on the floor with a child. Well, there's no way you can do that now, but it's a way of showing that everybody's got their own way, and Douglas could do that. I couldn't do it. You develop your own approach to children and it comes from your own thoughts. I think everybody can be taught a successful approach or technique, so you can certainly teach that. After that, I think some people are naturally more understanding of children.

Let's look at something else. Amalgam restorations in first permanent molars in children when they're placed at the ages of six to seven, didn't last long compared with amalgam restorations put in first permanent molars in later age. Bruce Hunter who was in the department showed that very well. Why? We both thought, it was the fact that it was difficult to control the child, it's difficult to control the moisture, there are many of these factors which come into play. I think that's the other side of paediatric dentistry. And there'll be some dentists who were plagued by that and would prefer a patient who has more understanding, more maturity and more self-control and lets him exercise his skills to his best advantage.

The end of the Edinburgh dental school

I became Dean in 1987; that happened at a very difficult time. I took over as Dean from John on the 1st of October and within a few days the announcement was made that the Dentist Register was increasing in number at an alarming rate and there was a need to cut back on the production of dentists. That happened within a few days of me becoming Dean. And that became an obsession then until I retired more or less in 2000. I hadn't expected that; we were working towards designing and developing a new Dental School and Hospital and that was progressing.

And then it was a matter then of responding to this need to reduce output of dentists in the UK as a whole, in England and in Scotland. That was hard work. In the end, a decision was taken to close the undergraduate school in Edinburgh and to open, after that, a new postgraduate institute. The process was difficult, and within a few years of the closure of Edinburgh, I could cite the actual references, but there was a recognition that it wasn't a good move and it had deprived this part of Scotland of dentists, hygienists, dental nurses, technicians, a whole dental force that was by then being missed.

Closing down a school is extremely complicated. The ultimate responsibility for that decision was the Secretary of Scotland and their Minister of Education, so that would have been Rifkind and Baker, Baker at Education.

They had a committee which looked into the matters in Scotland. It was difficult because we were not convinced of the transparency of the process. The Vice Chancellor was deeply upset by the way the decisions were reached, and the Vice Chancellor was a very mild-mannered, intellectually brilliant man, David Smith, and he was very unhappy and wrote of his unhappiness. The British Dental Association supported the idea of cutting and that attracted adverse comment in newspapers. I'm not talking about local one. The Times, for example, said that really there was too much lobbying and a lack of transparency going on. The process was unpleasant.

But we were faced with closing the school. Now once a school has taken on a student, that's the contract and you cannot, because of how dental undergraduate education is organised, simply ship out your second-year people to a variety of second-year courses in other universities, your third year or your fourth year or your fifth year, you can't do that. You have to stick with your students. So, the approach had to be that first, we couldn't take in students as direct admissions to the second year.

We carried on and admitted our last group of Scottish students, and as they progressed through the course, the school closed down behind them. That was complicated because you had to make provision for people who failed their examinations and needed re-sits, and failures are not always because students are bad; they can break their legs and fall off a bus and all those other things. So with each stage in the curriculum, you had to have a remnant that would be around for another 12 months. And then we had to ensure that there was always a consultant and a lecturer in a discipline, present as needed, all the way through to the end. That required a lot of organisation but, more importantly, an incredible amount of cooperation. The staff cooperated with that but it was painful.

The university offered a great deal of retraining, all sorts of help towards new courses. A lot of people were angry and very upset; others had found new careers. A remarkable one who was described as one of the brightest researchers that the UK had was very good on the genetics of dental disease. He taught early in the course and he decided that he'd become a goldsmith. And I remember going to Goldsmith's Hall to look at an exhibition of gold work because I was interested, and there was his work and he'd won a prize or two. Nevertheless the school closed.

A postgraduate institute was planned to be called the Centre for Dental Education and I was put in charge of that at the end and made head of planning. There were difficulties because the infirmary was having its own financial difficulties and said it couldn't continue with the idea of running a dental hospital; that was overcome. I did the planning and costing, one after another, until we finally got to where we went. It was difficult to persuade people that there was a need for an academic department and that wasn't secured until two or three months before the entire new building process began, but slowly the thing came together.

The difficulty was that the academic side was only two people. We had Richard Ibbetson and one other academic, and that's a very lean academic provision. And other schools depend on the mixture of teaching by consultants as well as academics, but two is a very lean number and I think that's the difficulty which persists. It makes it hard.

The Postgraduate Institute

I was asked to run this unit called the Centre for Dental Education. And that was the one which continued with the MScs in Preventive and Social Dentistry, which at least I could teach and do. I was due to retire in 2000, after the thing had got up and running. Richard Ibbetson was appointed in 1999, so we ran together for a year; that was an enormous impetus. He came from the Eastman Dental Hospital, and he got going his full range of MScs and other qualifications and which were amazingly successful in terms of the numbers of students that were turned out and the relatively small numbers of staff involved. That was a great success.

In those days universities nominated people to be members of the General Dental Council;, they were not elected. I took over from John Southam in that role from 1987 onwards, and I stayed on with that until about 2002 when the Council changed its constitution and way of working. There really wasn't a place for nominated people anymore; it was completely elected. So that occupied me for a couple of years. I worked mainly on the Conduct Committee there.

23. John Beal

John was inspired as a student towards children's dentistry and subsequently public health dentistry. He described his research into social determinants of dental health and fluoridation. He became a consultant in public health dentistry and described the battle to get fluoride in water supplies and the work of public health dentists. I interviewed him at his home in Leeds in 2017.

******

I wasn't originally planning to be a dentist. We had several people in the extended family who were in various health professions: nurses, pharmacists and so on, and I originally wanted to be a pharmacist. I was at school one day and there was a notice for RAF dental cadetships and I thought that might be worth considering. I applied but I didn't get it. However, I did then pursue dentistry and was offered a place at the Royal Dental Hospital.

The Royal Dental Hospital

I started in 1960. It was a fairly uneventful training. I wouldn't have regarded myself as the top student in the year, I was average, I guess. I enjoyed it and lived at home, so I commuted in daily to Leicester Square and the Royal Dental Hospital, now sadly a hotel.[125] The first year was at Bart's, where we did anatomy and physiology and so on. Then we moved across to Leicester Square, where we did our clinical training.

There was Professor Pickard, who had a posh voice, I can't remember quite what he was talking about but I remember him, in one of his lectures saying, 'And if it gives the appearance of bubbles, in fact they are bubbles.' he was quite a character. Professor Arthur Chick in prosthetics, and I remember very well Professor Walther in orthodontics, who was also a farmer, so you didn't see him on Monday mornings because he spent all his weekends away at his farm. It was 1960s dentistry, so we had all our chairs in a row. Sterilisation was in boiling water.

---

[125] The Royal Dental Hospital in Leicester Square closed in 1985.

After I qualified, I had a house job in children's dentistry and orthodontics but I became the king of root canal treatment of children, under 18-year-olds. Just basic endodontic treatment, I can't remember the details. I wanted to be an orthodontist and then for the second time in my life I saw a notice on a notice board for MRC, Medical Research Council, research fellowships. And I thought to myself, I've always been interested in the epidemiology lectures given by Peter James, who was a reader in children's dentistry. I thought I wonder if I might have the opportunity of working with Peter James doing some epidemiology and maybe doing a PhD as part of that. I went off to see him and he said 'I very much welcome you coming to work with me, there's just one slight problem. It will be announced later this week, that I've just accepted a chair at Birmingham Dental School, but if you want to come to Birmingham, I'll see what I can do about seeing if we can put in for a research fellowship for you.'

The leaders of Public Health Dentistry

I moved with him and Roger Anderson to Birmingham, Dr Anderson was his lecturer in the Royal Dental Hospital, we went as a group of three. He was the first professor of dental health in Birmingham. Roger Anderson soon became a senior lecturer. I started off as a research fellow and then was appointed as a lecturer in his department. That was an interesting time to be in the specialty of what we now call Dental Public Health. It was very much part of the evolution of the specialty.

The leaders of the specialty were Peter James, Phil Holloway in Manchester, Douglas Jackson in Leeds and Geoffrey Slack[126] at the London Hospital. John Mansbridge, from Edinburgh,[127] led that evolution in Scotland. The four leaders in England were those four. They became known as the Probe Stickers Club and they were great friends actually, and certainly Peter James and Douglas Jackson remained good friends for the rest of their lives and they often met up. I remember Peter James often used to come up to Leeds and stay with Douglas.

Fluoride research in Birmingham

My research was really twofold. The big study I did was looking at the dental health of five-year-old children in two areas of Birmingham, an inner-city area and an outer suburban area and comparing that with two areas outside Birmingham, Sutton Coldfield and Dudley. The reason for

---

126 For more on Slack see chapters 22, 24.
127 For more on Mansbridge see chapter 22.

those comparisons was really it was the baseline of the study looking at the effectiveness of water fluoridation in Birmingham. Birmingham had been fluoridated in late 1964. The level wasn't consistently up to one part per million until 1965, and we moved in 1967 so it had been in for a little while, but in five-year-old children there wouldn't have been a major change in their dental health.

So there was no true baseline, but 1967 was as good as a baseline in those areas. Birmingham was fluoridated with an inner-city area and an outer suburban area. Sutton Coldfield was not fluoridated but was a very middle-class area, and Dudley, which was working class Black Country, was non-fluoridated. So, by following it up over the years, we could look at the effectiveness of water fluoridation, but also the social determinants of dental health, and that was what my PhD was mainly about. I looked at gender, social class, ethnicity and several other social variables. I carried out my study over several years and got a PhD for the social variable part of the study.

Birmingham was the first big fluoridation scheme.[128] We'd had the national trials in Anglesey, Kilmarnock, Ayr and Watford. The Ministry of Health, as it was, had published the results after five years in 1962,[129] and later published the results after 11 years of fluoridation in 1969,[130] But, after the 1962 one, it became very clear, as it had been initially with fluoridation which started in the States. The first fluoridation scheme in the world was in Grand Rapids in the States in January 1945, they had monitored the effectiveness.[131]

Early implementation of fluoridation

The Medical Research Council had been asked by the Ministry of Health to send a delegation out to the States to look at this new technique of topping up the fluoride in the water, where it was less than one part

---

[128] See: Dental caries prevalence in 5-year-old children following five and a half years of water fluoridation in Birmingham. Beal, J. F.; James, P. M. C. British Dental Journal 130 (1971) 284-8.

[129] The Conduct of the Fluoridation Studies in the United Kingdom and the Results Achieved After Five Years. Scottish Office, Ministry of Housing and Local Government. H.M. Stationery Office, 1962.

[130] The Fluoridation Studies in the United Kingdom and the Results Achieved after Eleven Years Department of Health and Social Security, Scottish Office, Welsh Office H.M. Stationery Office, 1969

[131] A baseline study had been carried out in 1944 which showed that children in Grand Rapids had the same amount of dental decay as in nearby Muskegon. Grand Rapids was fluoridated in 1945 and in 1951 their six-year-old children were found to have half the decay of those in Muskegon.

per million naturally. They'd gone and when they came back, they wrote a report saying yes, the medical evidence shows its safety, the dental evidence shows its benefits, and recommended that we set up some trial schemes in this country.

So, the Ministry of Health set up these early trial schemes and they reported after five years in 1962 and it was then up to local authorities to decide whether they wanted to introduce fluoridation. It was a time before the nationalisation of the water supply, of course later privatised, but it was the time when quite a lot of the local authorities, particularly the big ones, owned the water supply and so Birmingham City Council owned the Birmingham water supply. They didn't have to go cap in hand to anyone else.

The medical officer of health had seen that the Ministry of Health had published the report showing its benefits; the Medical Research Council had confirmed the safety and so he recommended to the Birmingham City Council that it was done in Birmingham. The Council debated it, and they decided they wanted to do it. There was a slight problem, but it was easily overcome because Birmingham City sold its water to some of the adjacent authorities, particularly Solihull. Public consultation in those days was a matter of the leader of Birmingham City Council summonsing the leader of the little minor Solihull local authority to his office one day and saying, 'Oh, by the way, we are going to fluoridate our water supply in so many months' time. You've got two choices: you can either carry on buying our water supply from us and be fluoridated, or search for someone else to supply your water.' And Solihull were quite happy with that. They had seen the reports and supported it anyway. That was consultation in those days.

The policy was implemented and the follow up to my PhD was monitoring the effectiveness. Over the next few years there were several local authorities who decided, even though they didn't own the water supply directly, to start new schemes. Newcastle was one of the big ones, a bit after Birmingham, but I think they celebrate 50 years in 2018[132]. Parts of Huddersfield were fluoridated, Scunthorpe and other parts of Lincolnshire, Bedfordshire, small areas in the Lake District and elsewhere in the country, were fluoridated.[133]

In 1974, the responsibility for making a decision on fluoridation passed from the local authorities to the NHS, and really the only place in

---

[132] The interview was in 2017.
[133] See John Bayes about fluoridation in Lincoln. Chapter 12.

the country where very much progress was made over the next few years was in the West Midlands. Birmingham was already fluoridated, but the Black Country in particular had poor dental health and again my surveys in Dudley, amongst others, pointed to the poor state of dental health in the Black Country. Several of the local authorities were involved in deciding. There was Dudley, Walsall, Wolverhampton and I think there was one more. It became a game almost because at any one time we had three of the authorities in favour and one which wasn't and eventually we managed to get all four of them to agree at the same time and the Black Country became fluoridated.

Interestingly, part of the follow up to my PhD was looking at Solihull, which by 1974 had come into Birmingham. The water supply went to parts of Sutton Coldfield, but not most of Sutton Coldfield. And there was one road in particular where the houses on one side of the road got fluoridated water but the houses on the other side of the road didn't and you could actually tell which side of the road the children lived on by the state of their dentition; it was quite remarkable.

One of the interesting side effects of fluoridating the Black Country was the teaching of children's dentistry at Birmingham Dental School. After Birmingham had been fluoridated the caries rate in Birmingham fell so much that they were finding it difficult to find enough children for teaching children's dentistry and they actually had to ship the students out to Wolverhampton and the Black Country for them to get experience of treating children with rampant caries. But of course, that ended when the Black Country fluoridated.

The battle for fluoride

In 1974 it went to health authorities, and health authorities do not make decisions quickly and, apart from in the West Midlands, they didn't increase fluoridation very much.

Then we had the court case in Scotland where Mrs McColl, a Glaswegian pensioner, took the water undertaker, which was the Strathclyde Regional Council, to court. They had decided they were going to fluoridate the water supply in Glasgow and Mrs McColl, who didn't have any of her own teeth anyhow, decided she didn't want her water supply to be fluoridated so she took them to court on legal aid, because she didn't have any money. That was the lengthiest and most costly court case in Scottish legal history. Many expert witnesses were called on both sides.

I remember Professor John Murray was one of the expert witnesses in favour of fluoridation as was Professor Douglas Jackson from Leeds and they shipped over some of the anti-fluoridation people from the States to give evidence and the Judge Lord Jauncey, who I think actually had a scientific background before he took up law, eventually gave his judgment. And he said, 'I am convinced that the evidence is very clear that fluoridation is effective; I am convinced by the evidence that fluoridation is safe, I accept that there is some slight discolouration of the teeth but that is not a serious concern and is not a concern at all to the owners of those teeth but,' he said, 'In my reading of the law it is ultra vires; there is nothing in law which allows the water undertakers to fluoridate the water.'

That put the Department of Health in England in a slight quandary because although it was Scottish law and therefore didn't pertain to England the legal situation was the same in England. Basically, what they said was, if it didn't work or wasn't safe, we wouldn't want it, but if it's just a matter of an interpretation of the law let's clarify the law. And so, we had the 1985 water fluoridation act which said explicitly water undertakers may fluoridate the water.

Unfortunately, that word 'may' proved to be a major hurdle because across the country, I think about 60 health authorities went through the consultation process which had then been laid down as a statutory process for deciding, and asked the water undertaker to carry it out by which time the water undertakers had been privatised.

So here in Leeds it was Yorkshire Water. All the health authorities in Yorkshire said, 'Will you fluoridate the water, please?' Yorkshire Water said, 'No, we don't have to. We may, but that implies we may not if we don't want to, so we don't think we'll do it.' That led to judicial review up in the northeast where the health authorities sought judicial review from Northumbrian Water who took exactly the same stance. They were already carrying out quite a lot of water fluoridation in their patch in Newcastle and Gateshead and parts of Northumberland but they then were saying, 'We don't have to.' And it went to judicial review. The Judge said, 'Yes, the water undertaker is right. The word 'may' implies they may not if they don't want to and therefore if they decide not to, there's nothing that can make them do it.'

So the government then had to act again. Tessa Jowell was the minister of public health. She said, 'The law is a mess,' they were her words. But the government took the water industry act 1991 and they changed the word 'may' to 'shall': the water undertaker 'shall' fluoridate if the health authorities have gone through the statutory consultation, have asked the water undertaker to do it as long as it's technically possible and they of course are getting paid to do it. It's a NHS decision. The NHS will pay and the water undertaker can make a small profit out of doing it then they shall do it. And that is the law as it stands now except that the decision making has now passed to the local authorities.

I hope local authorities will decide rather more quickly than the NHS, which were very dilatory about deciding. And at the moment Hull City Council has been through the process of asking for a feasibility study from Yorkshire Water, they have been assured that it is technically possible; they have been told of at least two options which fluoridate a larger or a smaller part of the city of Hull and, depending on which of the options, a larger or smaller number of people outside Hull and the East Riding of Yorkshire will benefit from fluoride. Hull City Council will next year be deciding whether to go out to public consultation.[134] They will have to do that with the East Riding of Yorkshire, who have several residents involved and they will go through a three-month consultation process. There are other areas of the country which are now looking at the possibility of water fluoridation and interestingly, the newly elected Mayor of Greater Manchester Andy Burnham is a past vice president of the British Fluoridation Society. He resigned from that position when he became Secretary for Health, not because he doesn't agree with water fluoridation, but because it could have been alleged that there was a conflict of interest if he was still a vice president. But he's very much in support of water fluoridation, so we're hoping that he might persuade the local authorities across greater Manchester to fluoridate.

To be honest, we don't need fluoridation everywhere. I mean the leafy suburbs of Surrey have good dental health, the inner-city areas of Hull or the inner-city areas come to that of Leeds or Wakefield or Bradford could jolly well do with fluoridation.

Fluoride toothpaste trial

The other thing which we were all involved with, Professor Peter James, Dr Roger Anderson and myself, was one of the big early fluoride toothpaste investigations with Procter & Gamble on Crest toothpaste. We carried that out in schools in Shropshire with two big vans, one of which was a self-drive mobile dental unit and the other was a towable caravan. We went out to schools in Shropshire.

---

[134] John was speaking in 2017. By 2022 no decision had been taken.

Professor James and Roger Anderson did the clinical examinations, and I did the X-rays. Now we wouldn't be allowed to X-ray children purely for epidemiological purposes, but there were no ethics committees in those days, and I'm sure, anyhow, that it was quite safe. It was low dose radiation. They were protected with lead aprons and so on. So we had both a clinical diagnosis and later when the X-rays had been processed, an X-ray diagnosis and I remember sitting in front of X-ray boxes for hours and hours reading X-rays and recording them.

Remember Your Teeth campaign

I was in Birmingham for ten years and, although I thoroughly enjoyed my time there, it was time to move on. And then I was approached by a Dental Public Health colleague, Tom Dowell, who was the Area Dental Officer in Birmingham, who said that the British Dental Association were setting up a project looking at and evaluating a dental health education campaign fronted by the trade association of the major toothpaste manufacturers. It was basically Macleans, that was Beecham's, Colgate, Procter & Gamble and Unilever, which was Gibbs. And so I applied for the job of director of the 'Remember Your Teeth' campaign and got the job.

I moved down to Bristol for three years to undertake that campaign, and again, that was really great fun. Technically, I was a senior dental officer within Avon Area Health Authority Community Dental Service, but in fact, I was seconded wholly to work on the Remember Your Teeth campaign. There were all sorts of interesting things about working with public relations people. It was a three-year project.

Area Dental Officer

At the end of the three years, it just so happened that the Area Dental Officer for Birmingham, who was in fact an oral surgeon, Ivor Whitehead, decided he didn't much like that job and wanted to go back into clinical dentistry in the hospital service. So they advertised the Birmingham Area Dental Officer job, and I applied and got that job.

When I moved back to Birmingham again, I was employed by the NHS but with an honorary academic appointment in Birmingham. So I've always straddled that divide between the NHS and academia, which has made my career much more interesting than if it had just been one or the other.

The Area Dental Officer was at the peak of dentistry being a senior part of the NHS. Up to 1974, local authorities had had a Chief Dental Officer who was very much a second in line to the old-style Medical

Officer of Health. In the 1974 reorganisation, the 'Grey Book', as it was called, set out the rules of who was to be appointed to the newly formed health authorities, and what their roles were. And although the Area Dental Officer was not a formal member of the team like the Area Medical Officer, he was invited to all the meetings of the Area Management Team and would decide which meetings to go to and which not to bother with.

So dentistry was there at the table. When budgets, for instance, were being discussed, dentistry wasn't overlooked, and we could ensure, as far as possible, a reasonable share of the money and the facilities. Sadly, I have to say, over the years since, the position of dentistry has got whittled away. Now, it has much a more junior role within the structures.

First, my work involved managing the Community Dental Service. I had two budgets when I was in Birmingham; one was a budget of about three quarters of a million pounds for the Community Dental Service. It was a big service with several clinics and a lot of staff. I also had a budget for water fluoridation, which I seem to remember was something like 45,000 pounds. It was certainly under 100,000 pounds as against the Community Dental Service budget of three quarters of a million. I had no doubt which one of those two budgets actually did most to improve the dental health of the population of Birmingham and it was my little budget rather than my big one.

I was a member, by invitation, of the Area Management Team, so I used to go to a lot of their meetings and it was really just making sure they didn't forget dentistry. They probably got fed up with me. The Area Pharmaceutical Officer was in very much the same position.

I also had a role at the dental hospital. I was a lecturer in Dental Public Health; I gave lectures. I was also the person responsible for setting up the in-service training and the postgraduate education for community dental staff across the West Midlands region. I had that role for the time that I was the Area Dental Officer there.

The Community Dental Service changed its name around 1974 with the new structure of the NHS. It had been the School Dental Service, but it was also the maternity and child welfare dental service, although it was never referred to in those terms. Just following that re-organisation, it became the Community Dental Service but was still very much children orientated.

I guess into the 1980s it continued to have a role in treating children but also an increasing role in treating patients who could not get treatment within the general dental services often because they were special needs patients and it may have been mental disability or some other form of disability which made it inappropriate or less easy to get treatment within the general dental services.

By that stage I didn't do any clinical work; that was my choice but some of my colleagues did. I found that once I really got into Dental Public Health I enjoyed that so much more than the clinical work, that the whole of my time was spent in the managerial, advisory and teaching bit.

The end of the Area Health Authorities

I was Area Dental Officer until the next reorganisation. I have never counted, but I have been told by colleagues who did count that I and my colleagues went through 14 reorganisations of the NHS in our time, some of them fairly minor but some of them very major.

In 1983 there was a major reorganisation where the old Area Health Authorities were carved up. Area Health Authorities were in two types. Some of them were single district Area Health Authorities and they remained; they were just renamed District Health Authorities. But big areas like Birmingham, Leeds and Avon were multi-district so the overall strategy was determined at the Area level, the big county or big city level. The management of the hospitals was at a local level, the smaller district general hospital level. Birmingham had five districts. Birmingham Area Health Authority (teaching) was a five district Area Health Authority. In the 1983 reorganisation, it split up into five District Health Authorities and they were all fiercely independent and so I actually ended up with one fifth of my job. This is the government's way of saving money to replace one person with five!

The rationale behind removing the Area Dental Officers was to bring the decision making at a more local level, I think. Over the years I have worked with and for health authorities or whatever they're called at various times, Leeds was a single health authority, then divided into two health authorities, and is currently divided into three health authorities. With the introduction of Clinical Commissioning Groups, Leeds was divided into five. Now we have three Clinical Commissioning Groups in Leeds and at the moment the proposal is that come next April it will be back to one.[135] The Health Authority by another name; the politicians will keep tinkering.

When the Area Health Authorities were disbanded, the five districts within Birmingham became District Health Authorities, I ended up with one fifth of my job. Leeds, on the other hand, was only divided into two districts and they, unlike Birmingham, who each wanted their own District Dental Officer, said we will share a District Dental Officer. They were the embryo consultants in Dental Public Health. It was renamed and reappointed after the interview process as Consultant in Dental Public Health and shortly after that the specialty was formally recognised.

I've always been of the view that one Leeds health authority, whatever it's called, is really the best level to make strategic planning decisions. The hospitals are going to make their own decisions about the internal matters, but the strategic planning of health services across a single city like Leeds or Birmingham are, it seems to me, best made at a city level. We've got one city council, and one health authority. The city council is responsible for social care and the NHS is responsible for health care, but increasingly they are working together and have to work together. People don't fit neatly into social care or health care. It is all part of looking after the individual and to have the strategic decisions made at the same level seems the most sensible arrangement. So, I'm in support of Leeds going back to one clinical commissioning group. That makes sense. But no doubt the politicians will split it up again.

One disadvantage of getting rid of the Area Health Authorities was moving away from the 'Grey Book' because there was no longer that manual. It was then up to the individual District Dental Officer or Consultant in Dental Public Health to make their own mark. I was very lucky in Leeds, which was two district health authorities. I was the Consultant in Dental Public Health for both of them and I was lucky they invited me to be part of the Community Unit Management Team in both health authorities. So, I actually had a place at the table and I was also on the Unit Management Team in the dental hospital as well. I actually sat on three unit management teams. And I think that was an advantage to the dentistry because it meant we could make sure that what was happening on one side of the city the other side of the city and the dental hospital were all kept informed, through me.

---

[135] He was speaking in 2017. Clinical commissioning Groups ceased to exist in July 2022, and were replaced by Integrated Care Systems. (The Health and Care Act 2022).

I left Birmingham in 1983. Leeds was only divided into two district health authorities and agreed to share the District Dental Officer, as they were called then. I applied for the job and got a whole city back.

The issues within dentistry at the time were always budgetary. Things weren't as desperate then in financial terms as they are now in the NHS. It was sometimes just fighting for a bit of extra money for dentistry rather than trying to safeguard what we already had. It was an area of some expansion. Although we didn't have the rules of the Grey Book, it was really making sure that dentistry was there at the table. I wasn't present at every meeting of the District Health Authorities, although I went to most of them, so they couldn't ignore dentistry.

I think this was to the advantage of the Community Dental Service because, until the so-called purchaser-provider split in 1990,[136] I managed the Community Dental Service. So, I could bridge the gap between the hospital and the community service. I think one success of doing that was that I could identify those, usually younger, members of the Community Dental Service that I saw were promising and would be good dentists and teachers in their future careers. I could second them from the Community Dental Service on one or perhaps two sessions a week to the Dental Hospital to do some work and teaching there. One of them became a professor at the dental school.

When the purchasers and providers split, I made the choice as Consultant in Dental Public Health to go with the commissioning side, but about that time was also the time which regional consultants in Dental Public Health, Regional Dental Officers they were sometimes called, were initiated. So I had a regional role as well and clearly to do the regional work and the commissioning role and managing the Community Dental Service was not really on. So I dropped the management of the Community Dental Service but continued to have an advisory role from the health authority side about commissioning hospital dental services, in the sense of new developments, outreach for instance.

I didn't have many arguments with my hospital colleagues back in the 1980s but there was one particular incident. There were long-stay hospitals for people with mental illness or learning disabilities. Meanwood Park Hospital was a learning disabilities hospital which closed

---

[136] The so-called purchaser-provider split followed the 'Working for Patients' white paper 1989 which introduced a split between those who purchased NHS care from providers. It was realised in the National Health Service and Community Care Act 1990.

in the 1990s. A dentist there had a very old-fashioned philosophy, if you call it that. If any tooth had got decay or was giving any trouble, extract it. It was very much an extraction service he ran. I thought this was not an acceptable level of service. We tried to persuade him to adopt a more restorative and preventative approach, but he didn't change his way of working.

There were other problems as well. He turned up late and left early; his sessions were not very long. Strictly speaking, one of the hospital consultants was his line manager; however, the consultant didn't do very much about this problem, so I stepped in with personnel, with HR support, and we did actually persuade him to leave. Shall we put it that way? The consultant thought I was interfering with what he should have done, but I only interfered because they didn't do what they should have done.

How did the purchaser-provider split work and did it work? I think because they were two new organisations, they both wanted to make their mark. The commissioners wanted to flex their muscles a bit. The providers were going into a time where money was becoming tighter; the pressure was on. I think they didn't work closely together, and they needed to.

The start of the speciality of Dental Public Health

There were specialists in community medicine and then they became consultants in public health, public health medicine initially, but when they decided people didn't have to be medically qualified to be in public health, they dropped the medicine bit and became consultants in public health.

Dentistry followed soon afterwards and District Dental Officers, who had to put their names forward, had to go through the usual Royal College of Surgeons' process for consultant appointments, including interviews with assessors and so on. But those of us who put our names forward were grand-parented in. I mean, there was no formal Dental Public Health training program. The first of us were grand-parented in order to set up training programs for the future consultants.

Not all District Dental Officers applied to become consultants. I guess not all of them had the tickets to meet the criteria. Largely this was experience and postgraduate training. I had a PhD; I didn't have an FDS although I have an MFDS now, ad eundem, so I didn't have to sit an exam for it fortunately; but I guess it's not too big-headed to say I was one of the senior District Dental Officers in the country.

The second consultant in our region was Professor Sonia Williams, who was an honorary consultant in Dental Public Health. She and I set up the first training program and although it was still possible for people to be grand-parented in we were training the next lot of consultants in Dental Public Health.

I think most of the people who applied had come from the Community Dental Service. One criterion was that they should have had experience in more than one branch of dentistry. Some of them had hospital dental service experience, sometimes just as a house surgeon, but others had gone further down the road. Most of them had some experience of general dental practice and usually more experience within the Community Dental Service. So just as the initial academic base the professors of Dental Public Health, people like Professor Peter James, that had grown up really through academic children's dentistry so that the early consultants in Dental Public Health probably had spent most of their career in Community Dental Services. But they were expected to have some experience of working in other services.

The founding fathers of English Public Health Dentistry

Peter James was a very self-effacing man, but his knowledge of the subject was encyclopaedic. He was very farsighted and set up the one of the first, if not the first, academic postgraduate courses and qualifications in Dental Public Health, the DDPH. The Diploma in Dental Public Health was awarded by the University of Birmingham. Right from the start he was developing the specialty, he was very good at bringing on young aspiring people. I had enormous respect for him. I worked closely with him and Professor Roger Anderson, as he became, for the ten years that I was in Birmingham.

He inspired me as an undergraduate. I found his lectures in children's dentistry interested me so I wanted to go into children's dentistry and orthodontics. He wasn't an orthodontist, but I immediately applied for a house officer job in his department, but he had particularly inspired me with his epidemiology. And looking back on it, I think it was that wider vision. Dentistry for the individual was very important, but actually trying to improve the dental health of a whole community was something which I thought yeah, that's what I want to be involved in.

Roger Anderson was very similar. He and I shared a room the whole time I was at Birmingham Dental School. Roger and I got on very well. We weren't in each other's pockets socially, but we did social things together.

I think we were the first unit to use computers in the analysis of dental surveys and that was back in the days when we had to write our own programs. We wrote in Fortran. We had to punch up the punch cards on a machine, take it up to the medical school four miles away and leave it overnight where it would run on a computer. The computer took up the whole of a very large room which was temperature and humidity controlled. Often we would go for a drink in the senior common room afterwards. We had to go back the next morning to pick up the printout, see the errors in the programs which had been identified and go back to punch up some more cards and then take it back to the medical school on the way home the next day.

Peter James got to retirement, and he was the editor of the Journal Community Dental Health for several years. I became his deputy editor and remained deputy editor for 25 years, in fact. But he died quite young. And I was a little orphan. I'd lost my two heroes.

Geoffrey Slack was older. He was a visionary, very much involved in the wider dental political scene and the Royal College of Surgeons. In fact, I guess it was probably Geoffrey Slack who got the specialty off the ground because he had those Royal College of Surgeons' contacts. He was a great person in the specialty's introduction. He wrote the book and Peter James and I wrote a chapter in that book.[137] One of my abiding memories of Geoffrey was as an external examiner at Birmingham and he was sitting in our room with Roger Anderson and myself one day and he suddenly reached into his pocket and he took out a diary, and it was quite a big fat diary, and he flicked through the pages and said, 'This is a five-year diary. That's the date I retire.' And I always remember he'd marked it down five years before he knew when he was going to retire.

Many of the original public health dentists started as children's dentists. I can't remember Geoffrey Slack's initial specialism. I think he was one of these generic consultant dental surgeons. Certainly the other ones, Douglas Jackson from Leeds, Peter James from Birmingham and Phil Holloway from Manchester were all children's dentists.

Phil Holloway, again, had that sort of broader vision. I obviously knew Phil from contacts within the developing specialty from an early stage in my career, and he had research fellows and lecturers working with him as I progressed. But the first time I really worked more closely

---

[137] Slack GL & Burt BA. Dental Public Health: Introduction to Community Dentistry 1974.

with him was when he was the chair of the dental group of what I think was then the health education council.

Aubrey Sheiham was a friend of mine, we got on very well. We did several things together over the years. I think my views agreed with Aubrey's, but I didn't always agree with how he expressed them. I think he was usually right and even when I thought he was wrong, I'm not so sure over the years that he wasn't really right.

I remember in about 1980 some correspondence in the British Dental Journal where he was criticising the six-monthly dental check-ups,[138] and Tom Dowell and I wrote a letter in response to that saying that we supported the six-monthly check-ups and setting out reasons: gingival health and periodontal health and so on and so forth and of oral pathology checks. But since then, we've had NICE guidelines which say yes, some people need six monthly check-ups, some may need more frequent check-ups, others can go for a year, maybe even up to two years. And maybe Aubrey was just ahead of his time, but he was always controversial. He was always forthright in what he said, but usually he was right. He always expressed it in terms of black and white and I think often things aren't that clear; they're a fuzzy grey, and although if I had to go on one side of the grey or the other side, I would often remain dark grey rather than quite black.

I think the specialty of Public Health Dentistry grew out of that original Probe Stickers Club with a wider group of people and it really took a big step forward when the British Association for the Study of Community Dentistry was formed and that was led by Peter James and Geoffrey Slack. Peter James was the first president, Roger Anderson, again from Birmingham, was the first secretary but among other people involved was John Palmer, the Area Dental Officer for Somerset. He was very much involved with the NHS rather than the academic side.

From the time of the purchaser-provider split there were new people coming through the Dental Public Health training pathways. Certainly here in Yorkshire, and elsewhere, we tried to make sure that our specialist registrars in Dental Public Health had some experience of generic public health. Our specialist registrar was seconded to work with Public Health in North Yorkshire. David Lans our specialist registrar worked on prescribing patterns in general practice.

---

[138] Is the six-monthly dental examination generally necessary? A. Sheiham, British Dental Journal 148 (1980) 94.

But I think consultants in Dental Public Health fell into three groups. There were those who like myself took on a regional role and the regional consultants were all involved very much with the Department of Health and although, as I've always made very clear, I was not a civil servant, I did a lot of work with the civil service and we all had lead areas nationally. I had the lead, for instance, on prison dentistry and was involved in the working group, which wrote the strategy for improving oral health in prisons. So, one group had that wider regional and national role.

A second group hung on, if I can use that term, to managing the Community Dental Service and being on the commissioning side of the fence. I always thought maybe that was a bit of a conflict of interest and that doesn't happen now anyhow, it grew out, but those people who had always managed the Community Dental Service wanted to continue that role and some of them maintained that because they enjoyed doing a small clinical commitment. And the third group were those who used the generic skills which they had got not only within Dental Public Health but doing things within the wider public health field and took on other generic Public Health roles including a small number who became directors of Public Health. There's still one I think in Liverpool who is the director of Public Health in that area.

Dental Access Centres

I was involved with the setting up of dental access centres.[139] There were press reports of people queuing round the block when a new practice opened in Scarborough. People who couldn't get NHS dentistry queued up to register in a new dental practice and the local media picked it up and then it was picked up by the national media.

It was in the time of the Blair government and Blair was obviously under some pressure to say something and do something about that situation and he guaranteed that everyone would have access to NHS dentistry within the next three years or whatever. And so the civil servants then had to say, 'How do we translate that promise by the Prime Minister into what happens on the ground?' And one way they came up with, the main way possibly, was dental access centres which would be available for people who couldn't find a General Dental Practitioner.

---

[139] The Dental Access Centres were set up as part of the political plan to make NHS available to everyone who telephoned NHS direct. They were set up in waves from 1998 onwards. See: Modernising NHS Dentistry - Implementing the NHS Plan. Department of Heath September 2000. Also: What is a Dental Access Centre? J Morris, H Lunn, T Prince, J Barrow. Dental Update (2001) 2 58-59.

They could have a course of treatment even though they weren't registered patients and permanently on the books.

We didn't consider a dental access centre in Leeds, but I did talk to Tesco's about having one in one of their big stores in a large local authority council housing area, but they said they didn't have the space to do it and we didn't pursue it with them. So we didn't have a whole dental access centre, but what I had set up prior to that was an out of hours dental service. I'd been involved to some extent in out of hours dentistry when I was in Avon. We set up a bank holiday out of hours service in one clinic there which was staffed mainly by General Dental Practitioners and then when I moved to Birmingham, we set up a bank holiday out of hours service there.

I remember one Christmas Day I took in some sherry and mince pies for the clinicians to share after they'd finished at one o'clock. But the queue was out of the waiting room, down the stairs to the front door. I stayed there all afternoon helping to do the registration and looking after the front door to prevent more people from coming in; otherwise, they would have been there all night as well.

When I came to Leeds, they already had a bank holiday out of hours service but after a while we extended that to every night of the week and weekends. We decided we would use that facility during the day as a dental access centre. I can't remember how many years we ran it as an access centre, but then it sort of fizzled out.

I can't remember exactly why the dental access centres folded, but I think it must have been money. It was a time I think when the Department of Health was looking at other ways of increasing access for NHS dentistry and, to be fair, they actually made quite a lot of new money available. One of my jobs as the regional consultant was to work out how best to use the money which was being allocated to improve dental services. I think it was probably then that the access centres fizzled out as access centres and the money went into expanding existing practices or indeed opening new practices.

Professor Stanley Gelbier commented:

Peter James was Reader in children's dentistry and head of department. But from an early stage of his career, he was thinking outside the box. He was very interested in prevention and won, I think, a Colgate Prize to visit Scandinavia to see what they did for children, especially prevention, and their community approaches to planning services. Many years later he got me to apply to the British Council for a Younger Research Workers Interchange Scholarship which sent me for a very brief visit to Norway to see similar things, including their research. As soon as he left the Royal Navy James went to Dundee to study for the Diploma in Public Dentistry. Of course, at that time there was no Diploma in Dental Public Health. I am not 100% sure but I think there was a lot of microbiology and thoughts of prevention.

James later became interested in epidemiology as you can see from John's later account. He wasn't particularly interested in clinical dentistry but was lucky to appoint as his lecturer Gerry Winter, who later became consultant and then professor of children's dentistry at the Eastman. At that point Winter was replaced by Roger (Andy) Anderson, so the department became even more (what we now call) Dental Public Health orientated. James' influence clearly set John's mind racing from his student days for the rest of his career.

I would take John to task for including Mansbridge and Jackson as leaders of the specialty. They certainly were in the advance brigade for epidemiology, toothpaste trials, that sort of thing but if you look at my account of the development of DPH their names do not appear.[140]

John's account of the fluoridation events is excellent. He was in the thick of it.[141]

---

[140] The British Association for the Study of Community Dentistry, its journal Community Dental Health and the origins of dental public health: a 50 years celebration. Gelbier S. In press.

[141] See also: The British Association for the Study of Community Dentistry and the Speciality of Dental Public Health. Gelbier S. Dental Historian. (52) July 2010 20-31 and A History of the British Association for the Study of Community Dentistry. Anderson RJ. Community Dental Health. 1984 (1) 5-10.

24. Michael Butterworth

Michael studied dentistry at The London Hospital in the 1960s and went on to buy and modernise a practice in Suffolk. He was involved in vocational training and then worked full-time in Dental Protection. He spoke to Janet Heath in 2013.

******

When I was about 14, my father got a book out of the library about dentistry because he wanted to have some teeth sorted out. I looked at the book and I liked the pictures and a few words, and decided I wanted to be a dentist. When I was 16, I got a place at The London Hospital to start when I was 18, only three Es, which I achieved at A-Level. I started in 1965.

Personalities at the London Hospital

At the London was Professor Allred. I thought his insight into his way of going about cavity preparation was a revolution then. I learnt an awful lot from him. Aubrey Sheiham broadened my mind and made me think a little wider, Bernie Keiser got me very involved in periodontal disease, which I am still very interested in, and Professor Seward taught me quite a lot of oral surgery.

They were heads of department, or near the top, but fortunately, we could get one-to-one tuition, perhaps most of all from Professor Fish, who was Professor of Prosthetics. I suffer from a learning difficulty and I had great difficulty passing exams, and he took me on one-to-one and spent quite a lot of time, in one particular year, making sure I could pass the written as well as the practical. I had no problem with the practical; it was with the written. He didn't teach me any prosthetics because I had already done the course, but he taught me how to pass. Those were my influences.

There were 50 students in the year. There were five girls, and because it was The London, something like 40 of them were Jewish. I'm still in touch with a lot of those people. In fact, I still work with at least two of them. We've had reunions.

We started in 1965 and started the clinical course in 1966. And we were the first year at The London to have this new teaching method, which was devised by Harry Allred under Slack's advice, because Geoffrey Slack was Dean. That was small groups where you did all the subjects in a week. So you would have a morning of prosthetics, and an afternoon of oral surgery. And it was very hands on, so we were treating patients within a fortnight of getting onto the clinic in the first clinical year, whereas most courses were an extended period in the phantom head room. And to give an example, I've never, ever drilled a plastic tooth. I've only ever worked on real teeth; first drilling them, holding them in the hand. Within six weeks, right at the beginning, I filled my first cavity, I think in treatment planning, so it was a very different course.

There were minimal lectures and we had small tutorial groups, and Allred insisted we treated the patients lying down. We had the old-style chairs, but you learnt to treat the patients flat. And because I'm left-handed and he was left-handed, we learnt to treat with either hand. It was natural to take teeth out with either hand, which was novel. The course made me think a lot about what I was doing.

After I qualified I went into general practice. I was offered a registrar's job at The London but I turned it down, probably stupidly, because I've always had this interest in learning. So, I had a part-time job there as a research assistant for a few years and then I moved on into full-time practice, and later I went back to teaching.

Terrible School Dental Service

I had a very brief period in the School Dental Service, a couple of years. That was terrible. I was interested in it because from a philosophical point of view, I thought that preventative dentistry in a school setting would be better. Thamesmead opened a combined medical and dental clinic, which I think was quite revolutionary in its day, and I thought this was the place I needed to be.[142]

The first thing I discovered was that, although we worked in surgeries alongside each other on the same corridor, doctors and dentists didn't speak to each other; you had to write to each other, which was strange. And, I don't know why and I can't explain it, there was an inefficiency in the service. I might see a patient every half an hour in general practice, 15 minutes for check-ups. I would see one every hour in the school

---

[142] See: Thamesmead, Health Care and Community Dental Education. S Gelbier. Dental Historian 2019 64 (2) 54-60.

service and it struck me as very inefficient and as a result I got very bored. I didn't last very long; I was there a couple of years and then I couldn't cope with it anymore. It was tedious, to be honest.

Dental Practice

Then I worked for a chap called Dougie Albert in Redhill. He was on the Dental Rates Study Group and was a great tutor on the Health Service, so I felt that in the couple of years I was there I'd a great mastery of the Health Service and the background and the rationale to it.[143]

I decided, with my wife, that we would move out of London, and we wanted to move to Suffolk. And I ended up doing a locum in a practice in Lowestoft, a chap called Mick Watkins, who I think was vice-chair of the Dental Practice Board.[144] So I got another insight into the workings of that organisation. And through him I found a practice in a little town called Eye in Suffolk, which we moved to in about 1973.

The owner had died sadly, and so I did a locum there for a few days at the end of 1972 and I purchased it in 1973. The first thing I did was go through the records to see what I'd bought. And I discovered that there'd only been one crown made, which was a plastic crown. There were no root fillings done, there was no periodontal disease because alternate teeth were taken out if there was a Class 2 cavity, so it was easy to clean what was left.

There was a huge prosthetic element. The radiographs were sent to the local chemist to have them developed. It was very different from what I'd been taught and what I'd been used to, and in my early days I think I used to make something like 40 sets of complete dentures a week. But over the 16 years, we changed to a much more modern approach to dentistry, but in the early days, it was quite an eye opener. I don't know whether it was atypical.

We went through some phases rapidly. We quickly built up a waiting list and people were waiting for six months for an appointment. I was single-handed, and the waiting room was in the back room and the surgery was in the front room.

---

[143] The Dental Rates Study Group was set up on the recommendation of the Pilkington Commission on doctors' and dentists' remuneration (Royal Commission 1960) to set general dentist service fees so that dentists in the service earn on average the target income accepted by the government. See: The Dental Rates Study Group--a review of methods. DM Scarrott British Dental Journal (1979) volume 146, 151–158.
[144] Dental Practice Board See chapter 7, 11, 12.

The first thing we did was to convert it to low seated, using the conventional chair approach I'd had in the hospital. And then in 1974/75 we converted an old stable block in the garden to a four-surgery practice and we moved into there, and I took on an associate and a hygienist. I was probably one of the few practices that had a full-time hygienist working exclusively for me. It had its disadvantages. For example, if you weren't in the practice, she couldn't work. I think as far as I know, she's still there.

Obviously when we put the new practice in, we went low seated. We developed the practice and we dabbled in things like sedation. Everything was as modern as we could do it at the time; and we also got into computing, in about 1985.

Vocational training

I used to join Ken Horrocks at his vocational scheme in Ipswich, just for the pleasure of mixing with dentists, particularly young dentists. Then Ken was ill for a period, so although it wasn't official, I ran the scheme for him for a few months until he could get back on his feet. So I got involved, and I used to talk and give presentations.

We used to have the students come to the practice. We used to photograph them doing various aspects of treatment on each other, to show them how their posture was all wrong and that they were not doing themselves any good. Backache was all to do with adapting to the equipment rather than adapting the equipment to the way they worked. There were other things, oral surgery ideas etc. We did lots of different things that we tried to teach them and I got very involved in it. And obviously, as a consequence, I had my own VT, who was with me for about a year.

Moving VT from a voluntary scheme, associate based, onto a compulsory scheme was a huge change. I think it's an important scheme.[145] It's a stepping into the practical aspects of dentistry in a Health Service setting, from leaving dental school and you need something like that.

I was probably, 99 per cent NHS. I've always had this belief in the Health Service, and I always tried to do it. Now I think I would be slightly different, because I think that the demands of dentistry have changed. But in those days, we were still coming to terms with prevention, which

---

[145] It became mandatory to do vocational training to work in the NHS in 1988. See Gorden Fordyce's interview chapter 8.

was in its infancy when I first started. Repair was dominating everything. There were the great amalgam factories of the 1960s and they were still prevalent in the 1970s.

We were trying to have a practice where you didn't have disease, and that you took control of not having disease. To give an example, I was investigated by the Family Health Service Authority in those days for being one of the highest grossers in Suffolk on the Health Service. And when I asked them what the problem was, they said, 'Well, you've got the lowest cost per estimate, but the highest turnover.' And I think that was because, although we started off with patients with no teeth and dentures, when their children and grandchildren came through, we ended up with a cohort of patients who had no disease. And that wasn't to do with dentistry; that was to do with motivation. It was to do also with things like fluoride toothpaste. Those people changed from their ancestors and we'd got a practice where people needed little work doing.

Maybe we'd done all the old-fashioned work, the root fillings and the crowns and things, to stabilise patients, and we had people who were coming and they were more interested in their periodontium and whether they were coping with cleaning their teeth. They were interested in their children having no cavities and it was a very different style of practice from the beginning, which was blood and thunder and loads of dentures.

Later I got a job at The London, teaching treatment planning for half a day, and then doing half a day in research, and I got very interested in periodontal disease.

Medical protection

Then I decided I'd like to get a job with the Medical Protection Society. I put a locum in the practice and went to work with them full-time, which was a bit dangerous because I was selling it at the time. Perhaps from a business point of view it was not the best decision, but I became obsessed with my work and I had to go to London, five hours commuting a day for three years, and then we bought a flat in London for Monday to Friday use. I worked very long hours, I think anybody who works with protection organisations will say, 'People don't realise the long hours that you work and the nights away.' It was very intensive.

I joined a team of three, so I became the fourth full-time dento-legal advisor. There were three part-timers, each doing one day a week, so it was a very small team.

A number of things have changed. The number of dentists in the country has grown, obviously, and the dental membership of the Medical

Protection Society, now Dental Protection as we know it, has grown. You only have to look at the dentists' register to see that. But perhaps more importantly, the systems have changed over the years. And now we have problems with the Health Service, but they take longer. We have problems with the General Dental Council as we did then, but they take longer. We have solicitors specialising in suing dentists, so it all adds to the work. And if I give you an example, when I started in 1987, we used to go to the Dental Council with cases for two or three weeks a year. Now, they run two committees consecutively almost 52 weeks of the year. The work and its complexity has increased. You've had growth in dentists, complaints, claims, and the amount of work in the Dental Council.

The other thing that's changed for the protection organisations is they've all moved to having in-house legal teams, some of which deal with conduct and some of which deal with claims. They have a number of people dealing with claims, who are legally qualified, and who you work in partnership with, the dentist advising on the dentistry and its influence on the legal aspects, and the lawyer, interested in the dentistry, but looking at the legal aspects. It's become a complex science now.

The types of treatment have changed. Whereas when I started, we used to get a lot of complaints about dentures, complaints about single crowns not working properly, fewer complaints about endodontics. Now we get a lot of complaints about endodontics, about aesthetic work of one form or another, veneers, crowns, bleaching. And about value for money, a lot of implant-related work, things like paraesthesia, minor oral surgery, have always been there and will always be there.

I think money, both in the Health Service and privately, has driven complaints over the years, because of people's expectations. And if you remember, we had the Patients' Charter about 25 years ago, and I think from then onwards patients were paying more and more on the Health Service and complaining more. So now you can pay hundreds of pounds. You'll remember the days when we started where patients put £1.50 on the table and that was it. I think there's a direct link between the amount they pay, and it follows therefore that when they pay privately, they're expecting value for money. And I think also with the advent of aesthetic dentistry, crowns, bridges, veneers in particular, bleaching, etc, people are paying large sums of money, some of them money which you can equate to small cars, and therefore when the goods don't meet the expectation, it starts a complaint.

Under the Pre-Action Protocols that came in, I think it was 1990, you have to explore a claim before it goes to court. Because of the way the patients' lawyers get paid, the way in which claims are conducted has changed dramatically. So what happens is that the lawyers sift out the cases that they think they can make stick. So, whereas when I first started, in the 1980s, I would be in court with a case every week and maybe one in ten we'd lose, these days it's incredibly rare to go to court because most of the cases you're going to have to settle because the solicitors are on a no win no fee basis, and they are making sure that the case has been properly investigated. So that when we eventually get it, as a letter, there will be merit in some aspect of the claim. We'll defend what we can but often we can't, which is why it's there, and therefore we tend to settle out of court. The number of claims and the number that are settled have gone up, so the cost has gone up as a consequence.

There are at least half a dozen firms specialising in dental cases now, if not more. And that half a dozen that I would identify have either had experience of working in the other firms, which started with dentistry, or having dentists working for them. There are quite a few doubly qualified dentist-lawyers working for claimants' firms throughout the country. And I think that, as there is specialisation in dentistry, there is an even greater specialisation in the law. There are firms specialising just in dental claims, and firms specialising in patient claims and personal injury, that they have access to panels of dentists, or they are dentists themselves, and are able to pursue the cases.

25. Eva Milburn

Eva trained as a dental nurse in the 1970s and went straight to hygienist training. She worked in dental practice, care homes and a prison and did extra training when the role was allowed to expand. She was interviewed by Malcolm Bishop in 2013.

******

At our school girls weren't really expected to do any sciences, and our parents were told that we were all expected to be teachers. A girl in my class brought in a leaflet that she'd found somewhere which described the profession of hygienist, and I thought that's what I'd like to do, and so I set about doing it.

I think you needed five O-Levels to train as a dental surgery assistant. You had to do that before you could train to be a hygienist because the training's very short. You had to know something about dentistry first.

Training as a dental nurse and hygienist

I went to Eastman Dental Hospital to train as a dental surgery assistant. The course was a year; you took hospital and national exams and you were expected to stay for six months in the hospital post-qualification and after that I went straight to King's and did the hygiene training in 1975/6.

When I was interviewed for the dental surgery assistant training I told them then that that was my intention. And as it happened, the lady in charge of the dental nurses was actually a past President of the British Dental Hygienists Association.[146] So they took me on knowing that I was going to move on to that.

I was lucky; I just applied to King's and got in straight away. There were nine of us; I think one dropped out later, so eight of us qualified. There were only about 500 or 600 actually registered at the time. It was predominantly a female profession. A lot of people just stopped doing it when they had children.

---

[146] Vera Creaton.

The course was very intensive and we were busy. We didn't have a break, we didn't socialise, we were working and studying. Sue Bell was our tutor.

First hygienist in the practice

My first job was in Hertford. I came along and the senior partner didn't really ask about what I did but said, 'Well, yes, that's all very well, but what will happen when you stop to have babies? Where will we get another one from? We'll be stuck!' He was not enthusiastic. However, he sent me patients and was very pleased with what I did and when I left, he was the one that replaced me. Each of the partners worked for a day a week in hospitals and so I used their surgeries. At first, I was there for one day and later two days a week. We didn't have a surgery assistant; we were left to it.

I was referred patients and felt very much part of the team. I had to do my best to prove what I could do and I think I was treated fairly, professionally, welcomed and given lots of work to do. I just liked the work. Towards the end of the time there, we were doing a lot of fluoride treatments, which went out of favour later on.

I had a lot of explaining to do. I was very young and so the question, 'Are you old enough to be doing this, dear?' came up often. Sadly, they don't ask that anymore. But a lot of them were very accepting once they saw what I was doing, and I'd talk to them about cleaning and so on. Some didn't, 'Are you here to sell the toothbrushes?' was another question, because nobody had heard of hygienists. I can remember a lot of the patients, even 37 years on, and they enjoyed it and they could see the benefit.

Periodontal surgery

When I was at the Eastman, there were postgraduates and they did a lot of periodontal surgery, and it wasn't very pleasant. Luckily, we don't do that anymore, not like that anyway, not the gingivectomies without the prior care.

I had a break of a few years and when I came back, I learnt to root plane, which we didn't do before and we're not really doing now. But the ultrasonics were not so good in those days. They were only 3k; now they're 25 and 30k; and they leaked all the time. But we did our best.

I had a son in May 1983 and I stopped working, as so many people did then. There were no agencies, so you couldn't do a bit here and there, which possibly I may have done had there been agencies available. Later on I did agency work, locums and so on. So, I just stopped work until a practice in Cheshunt opened. A friend of mine was opening this practice, and she said, 'Come along.' That wasn't until 1990.

We hadn't heard of HIV as such; it was all AIDS. We didn't know details and we didn't wear gloves then. I felt lucky to be getting out at the time. I can remember thinking, oh well, perhaps that's a good thing.

Our scope of practice was quite narrow back then, but we learnt all the time. Since then, I've gone back to training in local anaesthetic and impression taking and crown re-cementing and temporary fillings, all those things have been added on since. That was much later, though.

Dental therapy

The therapists had dwindled. They had mostly retrained as hygienists because they weren't able to work in practice and there was just the one school in New Cross where they were trained and they didn't have work.[147] That has since changed and now hygienists are being dually trained as hygienists and therapists and can work in practice and are being given more work to do. They are very efficient and well respected now. I used to feel like we were special because there weren't many of us. We had to work hard.

Dental Hygienists' Association

We had a strong organisation, the British Dental Hygienists' Association, now the British Society of Dental Hygiene and Therapy, which includes the therapists. Once a year there was a meeting; now there are regional meetings. At the last one I went to in Edinburgh there were 1,000 delegates in the room. So that's really pleasing to see how we've expanded. We have a magazine, Dental Health, which comes out four times a year and between those, a smaller publication with job vacancies, not that there are many of those at the moment.

Residential homes and prison

I originally worked part-time in practice, but the rest of the week I was working at University College Hospital, so I carried on working in a hospital. And then later on a mobile round, we visited about 140 nursing and residential homes and people in their own homes. And we did a lot of work caring for mouths and instructing carers in oral care. A hygienist owned a practice where she employed dentists and she worked very hard to recruit these nursing and residential homes, and we went and did

---

[147] The New Cross School for Dental Auxiliaries closed in 1983. See chapter 28, 30.

hygiene with the patients. We could then clean dentures as well as teeth. We would go and sometimes three months would go by and take these dentures out and you could see they hadn't been out for three months. The patients were so grateful; it was very rewarding to see their faces when their dentures were cleaned. And then we had to get the carers to include that in their care.

I worked in a maximum-security prison, and the best thing about that was the patients never said they didn't have time to brush or floss. Except some were not allowed to have floss because, apparently, it's a dangerous thing to have. I was very well received there; they were very grateful. Some of them told me they had their money stashed outside so they could have their teeth done properly when they came out, so they needed to look after them while they were in there. They also got some good work from the dentists in the prison. I worked with a dentist in Old Harlow and she got the job as the prison dentist. She was going in part-time, and she took me along with her. I'd go one week with her as her nurse and the following week I'd go on my own and do hygiene work.

Electric brushes were very poor in the 1970s and 80s. Then oscillating/rotating brushes arrived, they were very expensive and few people had them but now they are widely used. Fluoride toothpaste became available in the 1970s and floss and wood sticks, single tufted brushes and disclosing tablets were really all the aids available then. Interdental 'bottle brush' cleaners made a huge difference in the 1990s.

26. Roland Hopwood

Roland became a laboratory technician in the pathology department at University College dental hospital and then the Royal Dental Hospital before training to be a dentist. He described the method of gaining admission to the dental course and thereafter of setting up a practice from scratch. He talked about converting to Denplan which saved his practice from possible insolvency. He spoke with Pam Royle in 2011 and myself in 2023.

******

When I left school, I worked in medical laboratories and my first job was at University College Hospital Dental School, which had just opened; it was their new dental school in Mortimer Market, off Tottenham Court Road.[148] I worked in the pathology department there and the Dean at the time was Professor Profit. David Main was the pathologist at the time and I worked for him.

I worked there for seven years and then I got another job at the Royal Dental Hospital in Leicester Square as a senior medical laboratory technician and it was there that I decided I wanted to do something else. I sought advice on what I could do with my qualifications that I had as a medical laboratory technician. It was suggested I could apply for medicine or I could become a technical college lecturer. I decided that if I could apply for medicine, I could apply for dentistry.

Applying for dentistry from senior medical laboratory technician

I made an appointment to see Professor Profit at University College Hospital. He'd known me for quite a long while, but he was decidedly unhelpful. He told me that I would have to spend two years doing A-Levels. I thought there's got to be another way. I had the Fellowship of the Institute of Medical Laboratory Science, which was equivalent to a pass degree at the time, and I thought well why can't that get me entry into dental school? So that's when I spoke to the chief technician at the

---

[148] The new University College Hospital Dental Hospital and School building opened in 1963 and closed in 1996.

Royal and he got me an interview with the Dean of the Dental School, Professor Lucas, who was also head of the pathology department.

Professor Lucas chatted with me for probably nearly an hour and said I didn't need to do three A-Levels and thought he could get me onto the first MB course. He was so helpful, it was a breath of fresh air.[149] And that's why I did it at the Royal rather than at University College. He gave me a place to start in September 1972 at the Royal, doing my pre-clinical at St Bartholomew's Medical School.

In wanting to apply for dentistry, I suppose, to a degree, status came into it. An example was one day I was working in the lab at the Royal preparing slides for diagnosis when a junior pathologist came and told me to clean the blackboard in the tutorial room as he had a class of students. I refused, but he persisted and said he would report me to the Professor, and did. As it happened, the Professor backed me up. And I thought that's decided, I will not be servile. I was a senior technician. I'd got my Fellowship at the Institute of Medical Laboratory Science and I thought no, this is not on.

Becoming a mature student

I was married with a child when I left my salaried job to become a student again. I couldn't have done it if my wife hadn't been 100 percent behind me. We were both working; I was earning about £1,000 a year and she was earning a bit more. We went from that to a mature student grant of £800 a year, but they paid all my fares. Shortly before my leaving do at the Royal Dental Hospital I got a phone call, and I spoke to a chap at the London Hospital, who was one of my teachers when I was doing my evening classes for my medical laboratory technician qualifications, and he asked me if I'd be interested in doing lecturing one night a week at the London Hospital, teaching medical laboratory technicians. I grabbed that with both hands because it was extra salary. They paid very well, something like £15 an hour, which was good then. It was hard work at the end of a tiring day and there was all the preparation as well. I did

---

[149] It was somewhat out of character for Professor Profit to have been unhelpful to Roland. He was usually helpful to students with unusual or difficult circumstances. It appears there was some sort of rivalry between the two schools and perhaps he was unhelpful because Roland had moved from UCH to work at the Royal. When Profit was Dean at UCH he admitted a number of students who had been thrown out of the Royal for failing exams. He once explained that if a school was not up to training a 'chap' another might be.

it for about three or four years. As I came up to my finals, I had to reduce that commitment.

At St Bartholomew's I had to do first MB because I didn't have the requisite A-levels, so effectively I was doing three A-levels in a year. I passed that and went on and then did second BDS and then did my clinical studies at the Royal Dental Hospital in Leicester Square.

I remember my first patient, a denture patient. He was a nice old boy, and I enjoyed looking after and caring for him and he was very grateful. He brought me some girly magazines, which was quite funny. I felt perhaps my approach sometimes to my patients was probably a bit different, being older and more mature, I think.

My first conservation patient was a woman. But the second patient was a West Indian chap who came in on the emergency clinic with an upper seven that was badly broken down. I wasn't sure it was restorable but the demonstrator said it was with a couple of pins, like I'd done in the phantom head lab. But the patient said that he didn't want any local anaesthetic, thank you. Of course, I was pretty uptight anyway. But he didn't move, he didn't flinch, I removed the caries, prepared the cavity, put pins in and he just lay there and just let me do it.

Once you got started, you just got on with it. And of course, somebody was looking over your shoulder all the time, making sure you're not making a complete mess of it. And I finished it and he went away. My demonstrator was fairly pleased with what I did, but, God, it made me sweat. But once you get into it you become more experienced and you see more patients in a session and yes, it was good. I enjoyed the practical side of it.

Some of the outside demonstrators, the people that came in from general practice to demonstrate, decided that they would set up a course at the end of our final year to talk about running general practice and such like. I think it was about a week or a fortnight of lectures listening to people's anecdotes, and that was quite useful. Another thing we did was to go out and work in a community practice in Wandsworth for a month. We were working on children in the community. And that gave us an idea of what it was going to be like in general practice and actually was a bit easier because you had a nurse who helped you.

General practice

I qualified in 1977 and registered in 1978 and I went into the practice with Graham Bond in Hainault. I did consider doing dental pathology because of my histology background. We did talk about it, but to be recognised it was an awful climb up the ladder and I had a family and, in the end, I felt general practice was the way to go financially. I don't think that was a mistake, we'd been five and half years living on a grant.

My aim was that I would eventually have my own practice. I suppose a partnership was a possibility. In fact, somebody did offer me a partnership. But I wanted to have my own thing, so that I was not beholden to anybody.

I stayed in Graham Bond's practice for four years. There were three associates, a full-time hygienist and Graham Bond. It was a very good practice, and I was one of the second year VT, vocational trainees' group, of what was the pilot study. So, I had a day a week off from practice. I learnt an awful lot there.

I went down to Kent University for the vocational training day release once a week on Fridays. Before they introduced vocational training, there was no equivalent in dentistry to that in medicine, where they'd have to do a pre-registration year. We were paid a salary as opposed to being paid per item-of-service. It wasn't mandatory for new dentists to do this at that time, but it became so.[150] I enjoyed it because I found other people in the same situation as myself, were making the same mistakes as I was.

One thing about going into general practice was that I had worked in dental hospitals for several years where I could go to different departments, meet all sorts of different people and make lots of friends. And then in practice you are shut in your room with your nurse with patients coming in and out and I found it quite lonely. It took me a while to adapt to that. Going and meeting other people outside the practice on the day release helped a lot.

I felt there was nothing I wanted to specialise in. I did everything, really. I enjoyed doing crown and bridge work. I just enjoyed looking after the patients, they were all such nice people, looking after them as people and seeing their families. I suppose you could say I was a family practitioner. It was great seeing granny, granddad, mum and dad and the children and I found that the most enjoyable part of doing the job, the continuity of care with the same patients.

---

[150] It became mandatory to do vocational training to work in the NHS in 1988. See Gorden Fordyce's interview chapter 8.

Buying a practice

Graham's practice was really well-run, the administrative side of it was excellent. He was really good with his staff and I learnt an awful lot, not just clinically. I thought after four years, I'm ready to have my own practice. I went on a course on setting up a practice, with my wife. It was an excellent course, apart from the fact that they suggested as soon as you bought a practice, you'd put a deposit down on a Porsche.

I was a bit naïve; I went to look at places. I was negotiating for a practice in Bath, and we'd been negotiating for quite a while. We even had somebody making an offer for our house in Brentwood and we'd found a house to move to in Bath. Then I got a phone call from a chap who said 'I believe you're buying a practice in Bath?' He was the owner of the practice and it appeared that his associate had put it on the market when it wasn't his to sell, the owner was not interested in selling. It was fortunate, really, because I was not ready to have my own practice. It was naïve, and it was a mistake, but fortunately, it worked all out in the end.

Starting a practice from scratch

We enjoyed living where we were living in Brentwood. The children were going to school there. It is a nice town and our friends kept on saying, 'Oh, come on, set up here, we're desperate for another dentist, the town needs another dentist.' So I looked at properties in the High Street.

We looked at a place; the rent was reasonable and I went to the bank, but Nat West turned us down. My father-in-law spoke to a friend of his, who had an accountancy firm in Chelmsford, and this chap phoned me up and said there was a manager who owed him a few favours at the Midland Bank, he would get him to see me. So he did, he came and saw the house where we were living and said, 'Oh, there's no problem at all; you can have all the money you've asked for.' So they lent me the money and we set up.

I had to give three months' notice to Graham. He thought I was absolutely mad doing a squat. He said 'You're mad, Roland, where are you going to get the patients from?' But, I decided that's what we were going to do. We got the place sorted out, got builders in, put the equipment in, did everything and we opened in the May 1982. And I didn't have a day when I didn't work. Not a single day.

We had patients on day one. I had days when I would work perhaps a couple of hours in morning and maybe an hour in the afternoon, but I didn't have a day when I didn't have a patient. I had a nurse; I had a part-time receptionist and myself. We just literally sat there and waited for people to come in. And they did. And within six months, I was working full-time.

It was National Health Service. If there were patients who requested private treatment, then I would do it but I'm not into flogging dentistry, I'm not into that at all. Within a year, I decided I needed a hygienist because I couldn't cope with the work myself, so I employed a hygienist, starting with two days a week.

Within two years, I decided I needed a part-time associate. The hygienist and the part-time associate shared one surgery, and I had the other surgery. We had another floor above which I eventually converted. It worked well, we were incredibly busy, I was booking some three months in advance. There was a great need in Brentwood at that time.

Prevention became the main driver of the practice. We were getting fit patients and patients used to seem to like to come to see us. It was enjoyable, and we were very successful. But financially it was tough. When we got busier, my receptionist became full-time, and we employed another nurse, of course, to go with the associate and she actually worked with the hygienist as well. The hygienist did fissure sealing and topical fluorides, and so that's why she needed a nurse.

The coming of Denplan

In the 1980s there was a 40 percent cut in fees. The review bodies' recommendations weren't accepted by the government and our fees just went down. It was very difficult. I still had a part-time associate. We were busier, but financially we were just going down the pan. It was just terrible. You just couldn't afford to run the practice. I held on because I didn't want to become a private practice. I wanted to stay in the Health Service because I approved of it.

But we were getting to the stage where outgoings and in goings were almost equal, and staff wanted increases in salaries. They didn't want to stand still. And they didn't understand that financially things weren't that good. In the end, it was my hygienist Ann, who talked about Denplan, which had started, and I talked with my associate. We thought well this may be a way for us to go rather than becoming a private practice.

So, we got Denplan to come and see us and they did all the calculations. They said, 'Well how do you want to work, how many days do you want to work, how many weeks' holiday do you want a year,' and all this sort of thing. 'And how many patients do you want to see a year, because you're going to lose at least a third of your patients?' that was their experience. They worked out all the figures, and I thought, well, this is a no brainer. Looking at this and looking at how I'm having to work just to keep my head above water.

I could see two-thirds of the patients. I'll reduce my overheads because I'd be seeing fewer patients. I wouldn't be earning a great deal more than I was under the Health Service, but it seemed you could care for them better. And I just thought I'm going to go with this. And I went with it and in 1991 I converted to Denplan.

Virtually every patient wanted to be with me, but I just couldn't take everybody. But the patients wanted to be treated differently, they wanted to see that there is a difference in what you were doing. And I think they did and I think we organised it well enough. We increased our hygienist time for them and I increased appointment times. I used better quality materials, and we just spent more time with those patients. And it worked well, it turned the practice round.

Within a year, we were seeing financial improvements. And patients liked the difference, they were getting something better. I was sorry to leave the Health Service, I didn't want to do it. But in the end, it was that, or I'd probably have to close the practice. And how does that help anybody?

Then, as Denplan became more successful and we would afford more things, I opened up the top floor and I put a waiting room and a surgery upstairs. Then I had a full-time associate and a full-time hygienist. The practice then expanded and my associate was still Health Service. Then, in about 1994, I converted my associate over to Denplan. And she was quite happy about that and the conversion went well. We still saw children as NHS patients plus some of our patients who didn't have to pay charges, the exempt patients and eighteen-year-olds who were going off to university. We had a number of exempt patients who'd been with me for years and I felt well I can't justify just saying I'm not going to see you.

The surgery assistants

The younger dental surgery assistants who were unqualified went to evening classes. But latterly I employed part-timers, who were all more mature dental nurses, people who had worked as dental nurses and had their families and wanted a part-time job. They were all qualified Dental Surgery Assistants. I found that the more mature dental nurses were more reliable. My original receptionist became my practice manager, and I had another receptionist and part-time receptionists who were more mature ladies. The practice ran efficiently. They were very good staff and I think they liked working for me.

One thing we could do to help improve our prevention amongst the children was to have days where we just saw the children, and they came in on their check-up days We decided that we would have a theme and that the staff and myself would dress up and that we would have competitions. We'd have the hygienist's surgery available so that we could teach them tooth brushing, do disclosing, and that side of prevention. The very first one, which was on the 30th of May 1989, was Roland Rat, because at that time he was a very popular television personality. So yours truly dressed up as Roland Rat. And the children came in and they just loved it, and so we did it twice a year.

Cross infection

I think one of the biggest changes was AIDS, of course. I was wearing masks before that, but we didn't wear rubber gloves early on. It wasn't until all the stuff with AIDS came that changed that. Then we started sterilising the air rotors because before that, it was just a wipe with methylated spirits or surgical spirit. The slow hand pieces and all the other equipment was autoclaved, but you didn't wear gloves, but we did wear masks. Then there was that Panorama programme showing blood being drawn up on the end of a rose head burr and all that sort of thing. And the following day the dental companies were inundated with phone calls. Have you got hand pieces, air rotors I can sterilise?

Of course it had to change. We were fortunate that I had a room on the top floor that I converted into a sterilising room. But nothing like they expect these days. I never ever had a boiling steriliser; I had two Little Sister autoclaves.

First light cured composite

In my final year as an undergraduate, my duty was on the emergency clinic and a young girl came in who had come off her bike. She had broken both her central incisors. The demonstrator who was on at the time said to me, 'would I be interested in using this new light cured composite material, which was cured with ultraviolet light'? He said that I would be the first person in the hospital to use it, so I gave it a go. We sat down and had to swathe everything and I had to wear protective glasses and gloves to protect my hands from the ultraviolet. The patient had to have special glasses and of course rubber dam to protect her.

I then carried out the procedure, bevel, acid etch, lined the exposed dentine with dycal, and then built up the fractures with the composite material, using the ultraviolet light for curing, and then polishing and finishing. I think I did a pretty good job of this and she went away very happy. That was my first experience of using a light cured composite material. It was 1976 or 77; previous to that it had all been chemically cured materials. Subsequently in practice, I used blue light cured composite materials.

I never did a basket crown. I did a bridge preparation on somebody that I did first MB with and I did pin ledge preparations on her lateral and central incisor to replace the central incisor. And that was quite terrifying really, drilling quite large burrs into a tooth to put in preformed posts or pins. And taking the impression over that, it was quite frightening. But it went well; I made it myself and it was fine. I've never used silicates.

Other new materials

I used glass ionomer cements quite a lot in my practice. Not just as a filling material, but as a lining material under composites where you've got a fairly large cavity to restore. It was possible to etch the glass ionomer and then place the composite over the top so that it didn't have to be such a bulk of the composite material because there might be problems curing it all the way through the bulk of the filling material. I did more and more composite restorations although amalgam was still the main filling material at the time, when I was in practice.

They were always improving impression materials and there were porcelain veneers which I used quite a bit; they were a nice way of restoring teeth that weren't particularly badly damaged. And Maryland bridges, of course, using bonding agents to stick them to the to the teeth. I suppose in my practising time, I did quite a few Maryland bridges. That started off with the Rochette bridge, initially, with metal wings that had holes drilled in them and you bonded those on with composite which went through the holes. Then the Maryland bridge came in the 1980s, I think.

Early retirement

In 1998, I noticed a small lesion on my conjunctiva, it was black or blackish and very small; actually, my nurse actually commented on it as well. So I went to see my optician and she referred me straight to my GP, and then I was referred to an ophthalmologist. And they looked at it and I had a biopsy carried out and it turned out to be a malignant melanoma. They removed it completely.

I also had melanoma in situ in my lower eyelid, and that was removed at a second operation. And then I was seen every four months at St. Bartholomew's by a chap called John Hungerford, who was the leading authority on conjunctival melanoma, probably in the world at the time. And I went to them until 2001. I was going regularly every four months and then and I was fine for two years, and then I started to get recurrence.

I saw John Hungerford and he said that he felt that I needed to have the eye removed, because there was a possibility that it could become life threatening. So, I had a full exenteration in March 2001. And as a result, I decided that I would take early retirement. I put the practice on the market and I sold it

I was fortunate in that I'd had a very good financial advisor who insisted that I had good cover as far as income support and also a critical illness. So that really benefited us, claiming the insurances for income protection, and I now see the consultant once every 12 months or so. And I've been completely without a recurrent since I had the eye removed.

I was very fortunate in that I had a really good associate and he basically ran the practice for me. I asked if he would like to buy the practice but he didn't see himself as a general practitioner, he wanted to specialize and he's now a maxillofacial surgeon.

27. Robin Addis

Robin is from the seventh generation of the Addis family, which started making toothbrushes in the 18th century. He described the evolution in manufacturing techniques and changes in the industry. He was interviewed by Malcolm Bishop and Stephen Simmons in 2013.

******

We didn't invent the toothbrush but we maintain we ran the business making brushes continuously for over 200 years, we think since about 1780 or maybe a little bit before. We made a lot.

WWI demand for toothbrushes and subsequent market

After the first William Addis made his brush, the really enormous increase came with the First World War. A toothbrush was quite complicated to make, and it had to cost quite a lot of money, so it was very much a product for the upper classes or possibly the middle classes; but it certainly wasn't a product that the working class ever owned. But when the First World War started, the company was asked to make a lot of toothbrushes for servicemen, and they found that cleaning their teeth was very pleasant compared with not cleaning their teeth at all.

At the end of the war, the market for toothbrushes had increased considerably because of the servicemen's liking for them. I think there was a similar but smaller effect in the Second World War. But it was predominantly the First World War which enlarged the market a lot. I was told the same thing happened in America.

At the beginning of the Second World War, the company received an order for a million brushes, which apparently was the biggest order for toothbrushes ever placed in England. It was for bone toothbrushes because they were uninflammable compared with the then plastic toothbrushes which were very flammable. They didn't want to provide soldiers with toothbrushes that burst into flames. It was a big job to make a million bone brushes because of the amount of handwork that went into them.

239

Manufacture of brushes from bone and pigs' bristles

I'm of the plastic generation but I think firstly the bones were cut out from a carcass of a cow and they must have been boiled and cleaned up and then they were provided to companies like Addis. Then the ends of the bone, the joint ends, were sawn off leaving a hollow tubular piece of bone which was then sawn lengthways into about five different pieces, some of which were straight and some of which were more curved because of the shape of the bone.

Those pieces were then shaped, I think in the early beginnings entirely by hand with spoke shaves, and in the later stages, there was a certain amount of machining to put the basic shape, the neck shape perhaps and the end of the handle into the bone. But the handles were then finished by hand. They were filed and polished and they were tumbled around with an abrasive material to smooth and polish them further.

I don't quite know how many operations there were in making the blank bone handle, but quite a lot even before you started drilling holes in it. I think in the very early stages the holes were drilled by eye, which must have been remarkably skilful. In the later stages the handles were drilled by machine, but that's from probably about 1880 onwards. But for the first 100 years, the handles were drilled by hand and the shapes were sawn by hand.

The bristles were supplied normally from Eastern Europe, from countries like Poland and Bulgaria and later Russia. They came from pigs which have coarse long hair on their backs and on their necks. They have soft curly hair on their tummies, I think. No pig produces more than a few ounces of bristle and the older the pig is, and the more it's been given a chance to grow its bristle, the longer and stiffer the bristle will be.

It seems to have been a tradition in some countries that a man who owned pigs and who saved the bristle from his pigs to sell, would keep a bit of the very best bristle from each of his pigs as a dowry for his daughters. Occasionally, their bristle was made available on the market, so if any of it was around, you would try to buy because it was the very best bristle of all. There's not a lot of bristles on a pig, but there are an awful lot of pigs around.

The bristle then has to be prepared to go into a brush. It has to be sorted by length and it has to be washed and, in many cases, straightened chemically or with heat. And for a toothbrush, the very soft split piece at the top is usually cut off because that's not stiff enough to make the brush, the stiffer bristle nearer the skin of the animal is used.

In my day, which was after the Second World War, there was very little bristle at all coming out of Europe, and nearly all the bristle was coming from China, and this work was done in China. One bought different types and colours of bristle, already prepared in bundles by length. I remember we used to buy some bristle from Russia in the 1960s. It was called Gostorg, which is the name of one of the Russian Trading organisations, and that hadn't been fully straightened and the bristle had a natural curve to it. We had to tie up bundles of bristle so that the curves counteracted each other. And then they were put in a tank of some sort of chemical and there was some boiling going on and eventually you got the bristles out somewhat straighter. But it was a very laborious and expensive operation.

If you make an artist's paintbrush, you want all the bristles the same way round so that they all have the soft flag at the outside working end of the brush and with a stiffer root end in the ferrule. But in a toothbrush, you normally cut off and dispose of the soft flag end of the bristle and you then mix the bristles around so that half the bristles are facing one way and half are facing the other, and then you have an even parallel sided bundle of bristle to work with. So when the bristles are put into a toothbrush they are folded in the middle of their length and drawn into the hole and then the two sides of the knot have a fairly equal stiffness of bristle.

Manufacturing brush making machines under license

I'm told the company was always trying to be in the forefront of mechanisation, but a lot of that was before my time. I only know what happened from the 1940s onwards. Before the Second World War, the company bought brush drilling and filling machines from Germany. And there were four makers, Canis, Zahoransky, Sachem and I can't remember the fourth one. The machines looked very similar to each other. I think all the manufacturers had looked at each other's machines and copied what they saw. They achieved their end effectively by being mechanical. They had no hydraulics, pneumatics or electronics. They might have been driven from an overhead belt, but they probably had an electric motor installed and they clanked around effectively. But there was quite a lot of work that the girls who were operating the machine had to do.

After the war, one couldn't buy these machines from Germany and our company certainly set about building machines because that was the only way to get hold of them. We're not really discussing hairbrush making here, which has a different sort of machine, but certainly the company had a formal agreement with an American company to pay royalties on machines that we built, and we were supplied with drawings to do the job properly. And we built quite a lot of hairbrush machines ourselves too.

Most of this was done at Hertford. It wasn't particularly complicated engineering. One had to have a fair number of castings and other bits and pieces which had to be machined up and assembled. There were small foundries dotted around. It wasn't terribly difficult to get castings made.

Moving the company from East London to Hertford

The company – I think it was a partnership really not a company in those days – was moved out of London at the end of the First World War. It had been in Hackney in the East End, which was not a salubrious place in which to run a factory or to bring up a family at that time. I think my grandfather decided he wanted to come to Hertford. He found the vacant premises of the Hertford Town and District Steam Laundry, which had closed down, and he bought those and the site was gradually enlarged. The business was transferred from Hackney to Hertford over two years and eventually, the whole thing was in Hertford.

Eventually Hertford employed as many as about 600 people. We were certainly the largest employers in the town, and we employed a pretty high proportion of women because they were the ones who both filled and packed the toothbrushes. We employed a fair number of men too, but there were other businesses in Hertford like a brewery which employed men.

We found printers who understood our needs and could do the sort of quality we wanted. The toothbrush carton which was used in the 1950s and the 1960s had to be made really accurately because from the 1960s onwards they were fed into a machine that assembled up the carton and fed the toothbrush into it, so they had to be precisely made. We used a printer in Wellingborough quite a lot. There were several printers around further north of Hertford. I don't think we used very local printers.

Queen Mary's dolls house

My grandfather made some very small brushes to go in a doll's house, Queen Mary's doll's house in the 1920s. Apparently, he made them himself. I'm sure he had people who could've done it, but I think he decided that he wanted to do it himself. And this was in the early 1920s and I think my grandfather was very proud to be asked. They're about three quarters of an inch long and he found it very difficult to drill the tiny little holes in them and he filled them with hair that apparently came from the inside of a goat's ear which was the thinnest, finest goat hair he could get hold of. He made a number of these and kept some as spares in case he broke any of them. So, there are little toothbrushes in Queen Mary's doll's house which was finished in 1924.

There were a lot of well-known people and well-known companies that were asked to make things for this doll's house and a lot of people made some magnificent tiny little things to go in it. But the whole thing was done free. Nobody was paid for making these things, they were made by very skilful men who donated them. I believe it's in Windsor Castle now.[151]

Buying bristles from Russia and China

To buy bristle from Russia, we went to dealers or merchants in London who had connections with the trading organisations in countries like Russia; we didn't do any direct dealing with Russia at all. There were three or four companies who specialised in bristle and related things like fur and the very soft hairs used for artists' brushes. One I know has evolved by way of things like feathers into buying in duvets and other products like that from China. I think that's simply because the bristle market has faded away and they looked for alternative opportunities to buy natural products from China. But we had no direct contact with these countries.

The company always had an interest in quality and I think that's partly why the company went on for a long time. I think that each generation in turn was very keen that they made a really good product and even when we started making products other than toothbrushes, quality was something that we worried about a lot. And there were other brush makers who probably made quite good quality brushes too. The Addis family over the years has prided itself on doing the job really well.

Sheet plastic and the start of injection moulding

The company bought two injection moulding machines in 1939. The record says that they arrived just before the war began, so I'm assuming 1939. And they were said to have been machines of six-ounce capacity, which in those days was probably quite large. I think they came from America. And injection moulding was a really new process and not many people knew much about it and it wasn't helped by the early plastics being

---

[151] See Royal Collection Trust web site.

of variable quality, and there weren't very many plastics that you could injection mould.

So everybody was starting from scratch. They had to learn how to operate comparatively complicated hydraulic machinery; they had to work out how to make properly designed injection moulds to make the toothbrushes, and they had to learn about what plastics were available. The whole thing went into a stage of abeyance during the Second World War because there weren't any plastics freely available at all, and at the end of the war the plastics that became available were often army surplus stuff that really wasn't very satisfactory. But gradually decent, consistent plastics became available and by about 1950 I think injection moulding was a serious process for making toothbrushes.

Before the 1950s plastic handles had been made from sheet plastic. The sheet plastic was cut up into blanks that were roughly the same size as a piece of bone and they were initially handled like a piece of bone. They were machined, and they were filed and scraped and polished rather like a piece of bone. There was then an intermediate development which was really compression moulding the blanks in hot steel moulds on little hydraulic presses. So the blank piece of plastic was heated in this steam heated mould and under pressure the plastic flowed to the new shape and came out as a handle that needed more trimming. I gather that the company ran such a process for 20 or 30 years but looking back on it, it must have been pretty inefficient because although the press moulded the handle to an interesting shape there was still an awful lot of trimming and polishing that had to be done.

Once injection moulding really got going, ways evolved in which you could incorporate the holes for the brush filling into the handle, so you didn't have to drill the holes anymore and the holes were always accurately positioned. And then ways were found that you could inject the plastic into the mould in such a way that the handles were then separated from the other pieces of plastic and would fall out as a complete finished handle, and any other waste plastic was taken away and chopped up again.

Injection moulding was actually important to the company because we started just before the war; it was a process that most people hadn't heard of and almost nobody had such machines. It allowed the company to learn about a new process before other people really got going with it. And it wasn't very difficult for the company to think about injection moulding combs and hairbrush handles and then, in later years, a whole range of other products. We became quite good injection moulders and I think some of that goes back to us having started very early on.

Nylon and the Wisdom toothbrush

Some people abuse toothbrushes badly, they scrub them on their teeth far too vigorously and children tend to chew them and you can destroy a bristle toothbrush easily. The bristle absorbs water and becomes soft. If it's chewed or bent too far, the bristle will break and the brush will just become unusable. Synthetic toothbrushes which are usually nylon toothbrushes tend to last longer than a bristle one because the nylon absorbs a small amount of moisture, but it doesn't absorb huge quantities of it and the nylon is fairly resilient to abuse, but you can still destroy a nylon toothbrush if you set about it.

The story of nylon is well recorded. There was a very clever chemist at the DuPont company in American who was given the job of trying to find a synthetic fibre forming material, which the DuPont people felt was theoretically possible. And after several years' work, he produced nylon; I think in 1936. And the very first product that the world saw with nylon in it, was a toothbrush. Nylon filled toothbrushes were shown to the world before nylon stockings were.

Now DuPont had a fairly longstanding and close connection with ICI in Britain, so DuPont licensed nylon to ICI and ICI decided that the filament that they would make would be supplied to only two companies, one being Addis and one being British Xylonite. And we had nylon in about 1940 and launched a new toothbrush which was called Wisdom and Wisdom was launched with nylon filaments but, as there was a war on, it was very difficult to get enough nylon to satisfy all our requirements.

What amazes me is that nylon has continued to be the fibre of choice in toothbrushes ever since. There have been many new plastics invented and many of them make quite interesting fibres and filaments, but for some reason which, I have never quite puzzled out, nylon, is still the fibre that everybody chooses for a toothbrush. It's one that absorbs a certain amount of moisture; it therefore softens a bit when it gets wet; other filaments would have behaved differently. Nylon seems to be the right one.

WWII and making brushes for armaments

In the Second World War, the company was not able to make all the toothbrushes that it could sell, so there was a shortage of brushes. The company kept in touch with the men employees who went off to the

Forces. I've seen paperwork showing how they were enlisted and where they were stationed. And they were all told that on their return at the end of the war, they would be offered jobs, all being well.

But a few key men were kept back. The company employed a lot of women and it employed an increasing number of older, more mature women as supervisors. And I remember after the war when I got involved in the business, there were several rather large and bossy women, and I was scared stiff of them. They were very important to running the company in many sections. The company also did a certain amount of work on gun brushes. They weren't a sort of brush that the company was good at making, but we did a certain amount of it. And we made a very peculiar little brush with a wooden handle for cleaning the inside of periscopes on submarines. We also assembled bits of radios for Murphy Radio in Welwyn Garden City and it made engine mountings for the Mosquito aeroplane, apparently. And although people tell me I was batty, I remember seeing an aeroplane actually parked in one building on our site. How it got there, I have no idea.

Making the tools for brush manufacture

I don't think I would have described the company as having enormous engineering expertise, but we had a certain amount. And by the end of the war, we had acquired more engineering skills and had learnt some new tricks and therefore the men who were quite skilful engineers evolved into toolmakers making the injection moulds needed for making the toothbrushes.

From the end of the war onwards, we had the idea that we could make compression moulds and injection moulds for toothbrushes and hairbrushes and so on. Gradually we had a fully-fledged tool room and then, in due course, another tool room was set up. We were perhaps not the best toolmakers in the world but we knew what we needed for our own purposes and we made quite good injection moulds. And like everything else, the methods in making injection moulds changed over the years and, by the 1980s and 1990s, one was having to use machinery of entirely different styles.

Plastics used for toothbrush handles

The first plastic that we used for toothbrush handles was cellulose nitrate, which is normally referred to as celluloid. And in those days, it came in the form of a sheet about a quarter of an inch thick and that was cut up into blanks and the blanks were formed into toothbrush handles. But I think cellulose nitrate was a plastic that was unsuitable for injection moulding and therefore the chemical companies evolved cellulose acetate which was a softer, more pliable plastic which could be injection moulded and was quite a lot less flammable. For many years it was the workhorse plastic for toothbrush handles, but its drawback was that it had quite a low softening point of about 80 or 85 degrees centigrade and was regularly damaged by people putting the brush under a hot water tap. The effect was that the brush head became very soft, and it opened up so the holes were very wide and then the filament, the bristles or the nylon, simply fell out together with the little metal anchors that had been in the hole. So it became a bit dangerous, people were getting mouthfuls of filament in their mouths simply because they put the brush under a hot water tap.

There was then a movement towards newer plastics that had comparatively higher softening points and could resist pretty much boiling water. The company would buy its plastics from companies that manufactured them. If you bought cellulose acetate, you usually had a choice of two grades, one was a high acetyl grade and one was a standard grade. When you bought polystyrene, you would have a choice of three or four or five different grades with slightly different softening points, process abilities, and physical characteristics. And the companies who make the plastic will vary the properties of the plastic in the way they think their customers need them.

Marketing and supplying

For many years, through the era of bone toothbrushes and into the early stages of the plastic toothbrush, the company did what most other companies were doing; it received orders from chemist shops to supply toothbrushes and more than likely you would put the name of the chemist shop who had ordered it on the brush.

In those days, in the 1920s and 1930s, the company didn't have a brand of its own and my father became more and more convinced that he wanted a brand of his own. I thought he had decided that the name Wisdom was quite a good idea, but I'm told that it came through an advertising agency who suggested it as a good name.

The difficulty was that it had been registered already by a man who specialised in registering trademarks and then selling them to people who wanted them. It was a way of making a living, so we had to buy the trademark Wisdom to use it on toothbrushes. And as a bit of an aside, another not very good toothbrush maker in Ireland went and then registered the name Wisdom in Ireland and it became very difficult for us when we wanted to export brushes to Ireland because he had the trademark already. In the end we bought the trademark from him. But the trademark was bought, and it applied to this new toothbrush that was launched in 1940 with nylon filaments.

Plans were made to launch this toothbrush and there was a determination that it was the right thing to do and that we wanted to press on with it. But Britain was in the middle of a serious world war and Dunkirk had just occurred and it was a very difficult decision whether to go ahead launching this toothbrush at the time that people were coming back from Dunkirk. But arrangements were so advanced that they went ahead with it nevertheless. And it seems to have been quite successful. People liked the idea of the new nylon filaments which couldn't be bought in enough quantity because ICI was stretched and couldn't make enough filament. But it was quite a successful launch of our own brand and I think the Wisdom name was quite a good name, quite a successful brand.

Making the modern brushes

Injection moulding allowed you to make a nearly complete toothbrush handle in one process, whereas making a bone handle or make a compression moulded plastic handle still involved a huge amount of work to get the handle finished. Ultimately, injection moulding allowed you to stand by a machine that just opened and closed and out fell toothbrush handles ready to be turned into brushes. Injection moulding and plastics transformed toothbrush making completely from a hand craft to a largely mechanised function. I think the transfer must have occurred largely during the time of the Second World War.

When you made a bone toothbrush, there was a lot of very monotonous but skilful handwork, and if a girl tried to put too much bristle in a hole and pulled it into the hole and thereby cracked the brush open, the brush was thrown away and she didn't get her penny a brush. They were working a piecework arrangement based on the number of brushes they filled and it was very important for the girl that she didn't have rejects because she didn't get paid.

Making a toothbrush with 30,40 or 50 holes to fill with bristle must have been a tedious way to earn your living. The girls were skilful, but it was a boring way to do it. After the war, they were being asked to take a finished toothbrush handle, put it into one side of the machine, the machine then went through its cycle drilling the handle. The girl then took it out and moved it across to the other side and the machine repeated the cycle. That was a noisy operation, and she had to stand there moving the brush handles around, but it was a lot more exciting than having to sit quietly, filling each little tuft, each little knot, by hand.

In due course, the machines got more and more efficient. Instead of having to drill the holes, you just had to put the brushes in one side of the machine and then you had to stack them into hoppers so that the machine automatically selected them. Eventually, you could throw a box of handles in and the machine would select the handles and they would come out filled and packed at the same time.

Industrial relations

I think it's recorded that all the different Addis men of the different generations were themselves skilled brush makers. They reckoned they could make a toothbrush as well as their workers. The business was quite small, the brush makers knew the boss, and they knew the boss knew how to do the job, and I don't hear that there were ever serious industrial problems in earlier generations.

In Hertford, in my time since the Second World War, we had quite harmonious industrial relations. I think it was largely because the people who owned the company and the people who ran the company busied themselves by going around and finding out what was happening, by being seen, by people knowing who they were.

I think that the management of the company was seen to be honest citizens earning their living the same as everybody else. I used to walk around, people knew who I was, knew what I did, and they could approach me and talk about anything they wanted to. You didn't always know the answer, but at least you allowed them the chance to talk to you about it. I don't think that in Addis we had any serious problems of employing people. I think people felt the job was one in which they would be treated fairly. They might not be paid all the money they wanted, but they would be paid a decent wage and they would be treated decently. I think we succeeded fairly well because we were honest people, really.

Managing the business

My future was mapped out from the time I was born, because I was the elder son. I didn't get the choice my brothers and sisters had. My elder sister and younger brother went to university and my younger sister trained to be a nurse.

I was moved into the business when I was about 22, when my father went through one of his phases and decided that he was ill and was going to die. Had he died, I don't think, at 22, I would have been very much use running the business. The problem is that an elder son pushed into a family business is not necessarily the right personality or character to do the job. Previous generations of Addises had seemed to have been quite good at running the business, but I didn't feel that I could run a business that had become large and complicated.

I contributed as best I could for over 30 years and I hope I was quite useful, but being a managing director was just not a job that I could face doing. And the result was that the family had to face up, fairly early on, to the problem of how it was going to run the business in years to come. We started to employ managing directors that were not connected with the family at all, who were recruited from outside the business. I think that was a good thing because they were probably on average better than the Addis family. Even now one also comes across, in the newspapers, stories of families who have run a business for a long time and have had to rearrange their management at the last moment before the family finally disintegrates in argument. And we did it before the family got involved in arguments.

Well, I suppose we had one advantage in that my father was an only child and an only son, and therefore he didn't have brothers and sisters who might also have had interests in the business. My father naturally ran it after his father died. And it's not a business where the ownership has been spread amongst several families, which I think is quite helpful, really.

I don't think the family had great plans to make the business an international business. But it had a lot of steady export business, much of which got reduced as countries introduced their own regulations about restricting imports. And gradually, over the years, the company has responded to the difficulty of exporting by setting up small manufacturing businesses in these countries. Most of them have been little more than making toothbrushes for that domestic market. But they were set up with usually quite cheap and simple machinery because the expensive machinery was too expensive and too complicated and there have been, from to time, difficulties in supplying spare parts for machinery, and sometimes even in getting raw materials.

Almost none of these businesses have been particularly successful or profitable. They were never the jewel in the Addis crown. Addis never saw itself really as being an international company with a lot of international overseas manufacturing. And most of these small factories were in old parts of the Commonwealth in rather funny little countries, and they haven't been successful, really.

The sales force

The company had evolved a policy that the best way to sell our products was to be in control, so we built up two large sales forces and one of those dealt with toothbrushes and other products that also went to chemist shops, like nailbrushes and hairbrushes. And to keep the salesmen fully employed earning their living we gradually added other ranges of products to the ranges that were being sold by the salesmen. That became a policy; you had to keep giving the salesmen more and more things to sell. And I suspect they sold less and less of more and more.

In about 1955 or 1960 the company decided that it should make a toothbrush that was approved of by the dentists' profession and a questionnaire was sent out to pretty much all the dentists in Britain asking them for their advice as to the size and shape and the nature of a toothbrush that they would like to see made. And because of that, and I think there was a fair amount of unanimity amongst the dentists, we designed a toothbrush that was called the Wisdom Multituft and it had 45 holes in it, which is quite a lot of holes to put in a toothbrush, and they were densely packed nylon filling. It was a very nice toothbrush. It doesn't look exciting by the standards of modern brushes, but it was a very good workable brush.

In those days, we made toothbrushes with as many as 55 holes, which is quite different to the modern toothbrushes that we see in 2013 when I'm talking. Modern toothbrushes seem to have filaments of different colours and apparently of different textures and different layouts, but they don't make the densely filled brushes with 45 or 55 holes, which make good toothbrushes.

We got involved in a battery driven electric toothbrush in the early 1960s. It simply reciprocated from side to side. It wasn't as sophisticated as the modern ones are. We sold a reasonable number of them. They were popular for a while, but had little impact on our ordinary toothbrushes. I imagine more are being sold because they are widely distributed now and they are being recommended by dentists. They were bought in from Switzerland and I don't know who the company that made them was. I don't think that Addis has really had the skills or the money or the will to evolve itself into a company that could make electric

251

toothbrushes. I think most electric toothbrushes now are being made by extremely competent companies like Philips and Braun. These are companies who have a long tradition of working with electrical devices and know how to do this sort of work.

I think the result of this was that the overheads of the company built up to unsustainable levels just trying to keep control of all the things we were doing and the time came when the company suddenly found itself in difficulty. And that was about 1993; it suddenly found it was running out of money. It hadn't really foreseen this happening, and we didn't really know what to do. But what we did was we reorganised the company extensively; we divided it up into two sections. One was entirely to do with toothbrushes, and the other was to do with housewares. Products that were not connected with either toothbrushes or house wares were just disposed of. They were just dumped, really.

Selling the company

The toothbrush business was then sold to a management buyout; in other words, the then managing director and other members of his team supported with money from an outside organisation, bought the company and continued to run it.

When our business was sold, it was divided into two unequal halves. It was sold as going concerns and therefore the employees went with the business to the new owners.

The new owners were given the portions of the pension scheme that was attached to the employees that they had taken on. And we were left with a part of the pension scheme that applied to people who were already getting a pension and people who were within the scheme but had left the company. In other words, deferred pensions.

It took us an enormous amount of effort and time to tidy it up and to check everything that we could check, and eventually the pension scheme evolved into a whole series of individual annuities with an insurance company and all our pensioners now receive their pension from the Legal & General. It was a final salary scheme and over the years when the company made decent profits and felt generous, it would put into the scheme a sum of money from that year's accounts. And I'm very glad it did because in the end, despite the trials and tribulations of shutting down the scheme and the difficulty of getting decent returns on investment, our pensioners got all that they were promised and a bit more. I can look people in the eye in Hertford and say, 'You got your full pension,' rather than having to turn away and saying, 'You didn't get all the pension that you were promised; we weren't clever enough.' I'm not proud of myself, but I'm proud that the company paid all the pensioners every penny that they were owed because not every pension scheme these days does that.

In 1976 and through till about 1978 the company introduced an opportunity for dentists and dental students to write papers about dentistry and its connection with toothbrushes, and that was quite successful and it was continued under the name of the Wisdom Dental Health Award, and I think there were small monetary prizes for people who wrote good and interesting papers. So, Addis did, in that way, interconnect with the dental profession. And from about that time onwards, we visited dentists in their dental surgeries to talk to them about recommending Wisdom toothbrushes. It was only a moderately successful activity, I think, because dentists are busy people and when you go to visit dentists, you too may have to wait in the waiting room, and having waited for some time you may be told by the dentist that he doesn't find you a very interesting person to talk to, and you may be sent away empty-handed.

I think that sending representatives around dentists' surgeries was a very expensive and rather unproductive activity, but it was done largely in response to other companies doing it as well, but maybe that contributed to the high level of costs that the company then tried to carry.

The toothbrush collection

My father put together a very interesting collection of toothbrushes. Most them are brushes that were made by Addis, but there are also brushes made by several other brush makers, and they're there because they're very interesting examples of the designs and the shapes and techniques used by other brush makers.

Apart from three or four brushes that have got mislaid, those that remain, and there are about 150 of them, are in my house, where I hang on to them and occasionally look at them because they are very nice indeed. Some other toothbrushes that were around when the business was closed down have found their way to the Hertford Museum. There are several quite nice toothbrushes in the Hertford Museum and some not so interesting ones, but there is quite a decent collection of plastic ones, and quite an interesting selection of unfilled toothbrush handles which are quite interesting to look at because it helps you see clearly how the bone handles were shaped and machined before being filled.

28. *Stanley Gelbier*

Stanley was an academic children's dentist at the London Hospital and left the dental school to join the Hackney local health authority and manage its school and priority dental services, which after 1974 became the Community Dental Services. He later became a professor/honorary consultant in dental public health in South London. He was interviewed by Stephen Simmons in 2012.

******

In 1967 I was a lecturer in Children's Dentistry at the London Hospital and I was encouraged to apply for the post of Chief Dental Officer of Hackney. After the Thursday night I was appointed, by Friday lunchtime, all the other 12 Chief Dental Officers telephoned, not only to congratulate me but to say, 'Can I help you?' I think that showed the sort of atmosphere which was around, which was quite different from hospitals and general practice. Several people said to me, 'What are you doing that for? You're better than that,' which really places on record the status that most dentists thought of the School Dental Service.

Profile of dentists and patients in the School Dental Service

It was partly warranted, because there were quite a lot of dentists in the School Dental Service at that time who were dropouts from general practice where they couldn't earn a living. Either they never could earn a living or they were coming to the end of their practising life and their earning capacity was going down. But there were also several enthusiasts around who were really trying to do things which were better than before. At the time it was called the School Dental Service because that's what it was; it treated mostly children. 95 percent of our work was treating school children and there were a few preschool children and expectant and nursing mothers.

Issues of funding for facilities and equipment

I had 12 surgeries in Hackney when I took over and within a couple of years, I'd totally re-equipped them and by the end of another two or three years I had 32 surgeries, all beautifully equipped. The significance was that the School Dental Service, as part of the School Health Service, wasn't in the NHS. It was part of the local authority and depending on where you were, you were part of the county or, in my case, the borough. But the significant thing is that roughly 95 percent of my money in Hackney came from the Inner London Education Authority. And depending on where people might have worked, it might have come from the Surrey Education Authority, Kent or Essex or whatever. The significance was that re-equipping my surgeries was petty cash compared to the education budget. As long as I came up with a good argument, almost invariably I got what I wanted.

To help me were these other 12 Chief Dental Officer s, and we used to meet fortnightly. We'd have lunch and then we'd have a meeting and we planned together what we could get.

I was also Principal School Dental Officer. My home base was Hackney, where I was Chief Dental Officer. But they were only paying for something like five percent, not only of my salary but the cost of the whole budget; most of my money was coming from the Education Authority. So whenever I went to them and said, 'can I have this, that or the other, and don't forget you're only paying five percent of the cost,' they said I could have whatever I wanted.

Moving the school service into the National Health Service

In 1974 we went into Area Health Authorities, we graduated out of local authority employment into the NHS for the first time. On the one hand it was terrific; at long last we were being acceptable to other dentists. But the pot of gold had gone forever. Yes, a lot of advances were made after 1974, but the ability to spend a lot of money never came back, to my knowledge, anywhere in the country, not in the same way.

The salaries of school dentists was minimal. I can't remember just how much school dentists were earning just before the reorganisation, when it was negotiated by the Dental Whitley Council. But after 1974, when it was just part of the NHS, the salaries went up. And part of it was this new function called Area Dental Officer. Now, for the first time, dentistry had somebody of a very senior level, at Health Authority level, to represent the whole of dentistry. And that was agreed by the British Dental Association. In fact, they made sure the jobs were advertised and open to everybody in the profession, not just school dentists.

As a result, they had a large salary comparative to other people at that time. They also made sure that the School Dental Service was headed by the Area Dental Officer and that was the salary. Whenever you're negotiating, make sure you fight not for the people at the bottom initially, but the people at the top because in salaried situations, everything tumbles down. If the guy at the top is earning a lot, then the district dental officers, the senior dental officers and so on would also earn a lot. So, the whole salary structure of the School Dental Service changed.

Before the changeover, it was decided that school dental services would be inspected by the Ministry of Health. There was a compulsory inspection by dental officers from the Ministry every three years, and if you were no good, they'd come back annually. Just after I arrived in Hackney, I remember Gordon Potter coming from the then Ministry of Health. They worked jointly between the Ministry of Education and the Ministry or Department of Education. They were joint dental officers. Before he came, he would ask for all the statistics of the service. He wanted to know not only what the service was doing, but what individual dentists were doing. He had all this information, with his slide rule in those days, no computers, and he'd work out the average productivity of every dentist before he came. As Chief Dental Officer, I had to account for why some people were doing more than average and some people were doing far less.

I had said when I arrived that, although we had a big waiting list for treatment, we wanted to do prevention, almost unheard of at the time, in 1967. I was backed by the Medical Officer of Health, but the Ministry came down and thought this was terrible, spending time on prevention when you could be doing treatment. And they put in a report which really slammed the School Dental Service and the report in those days went to the chief officer who was the Town Clerk, who was a legal guy. I was responsible to the Medical Officer of Health; he was responsible to the Town Clerk. And I remember being sent for, with the Medical Officer of Health, by the Town Clerk and we had to explain why we thought we were ahead of the game, not behind it. And fortunately, he supported us and wrote back to the Ministry that they needed to come into the modern age.

Years later, when I was doing my PhD, rummaging in the Public Record Office I came across some of these reports and there was the report on Hackney, the one where I'd been inspected and Potter had said, 'Our new Chief Dental Officer is called Gelbier, and if he can do half as much as he says, he might be alright.'

Anyway, maybe that's given some thoughts whether things are better or worse after the reorganisation. Then one or two authorities were treating elderly people and the handicapped. Again, I had two surgeries for the handicapped at that time and again got heavily criticised because the Ministry said, 'It's not within the rules,' and the borough, thank God, said, 'Sue us.'

Further education for dentists

The School Dental Service and then the Community Service were ahead of all branches of dentistry in education. Chief dental officers, and later Area Dental Officers, piled a lot of money into education, both in sending dental officers on courses and also starting vocational training. The community scheme, based at the British Postgraduate Medical Federation, was the second earliest vocational training scheme in the country. We insisted it was not going to be just a few community dental officers going on a general practice scheme.

We had a committee setup of the four Thames regions at the time, and we insisted there should be a four-Thames vocational training programme, which took off in a big way. David Rule, consultant in children's dentistry at the Eastman was adviser to that course, I was the course tutor, seconded every Friday.

We totally raised the whole standing of the community service by doing that. And not only that, but made all the people coming from the hospitals and general practice aware of the high quality of the people in the service. It totally changed the whole picture.

I'd said before it was mostly a service of dropouts throughout the country. After vocational training took effect, it was the most highly qualified group of people. And I include the hospital people in that. And there were particular people. William Humpherson,[152] always made sure that lots of his people, not only were going through vocational training, but also teaching. I mean Les Cheeseman was teaching on vocational training.[153] Relative analgesia was one of the big things. There was a real hotbed of education when the first courses, the Diploma in Dental Public Health was started and it was started for overseas dentists, but several Chief Dental Officers decided that either they themselves or some of their dental officers went on those courses. Eventually, they became compulsory for senior people. Before the MSc started, everything was geared towards raising standards and I can't speak highly enough of all of that.

---

[152] District Dental Officer.
[153] See chapter 29, 30.

How things have changed since the early days.

When I did my first school dental inspections, I could stand in front of a class and say smile, and I could say, 'You, you, you, you, gas room,' because they had puss oozing out of all parts of the mouth. That was the situation in many school children in Hackney. When I first took up post and I looked in the drawer, there was a rule from the old county council, who were there before the Inner London Education Authority, and it said, 'If you have a gas session booked and there are fewer than 30 children on the list, cancel it, it's not worth having.' Yes! And that was more or less the situation in all 12 clinics. At least once a week, we had a gas session with about 30 children.

So, when people annoyingly say to me at cocktail parties or whatever, 'Nothing changes in dentistry,' well, all of us, in one way or another, have seen enormous changes. You would have a child, put a mask over their face until they turned black; sometimes there was time for a bit of oxygen to be added. The tooth, or teeth, were snatched, often many of them, you took them into the recovery room and they were dumped at the head of the queue. You had a sloping basin and they were all dribbling blood. It certainly has changed in our lifetimes.

In one of the earliest toothpaste trials they gave out fluoride toothpaste. If you say to people, use it every morning and every night and you go round to people's homes, you say how often are your children using the toothpaste and the brushes which we supplied, they'll tell you morning and night time. But what this person organising the trial did is he got the person doing the home visit always to ask, can they could use the lavatory? And when they went to the lavatory, they checked in the cabinets to see, and in several cases, clearly the toothpaste had never been opened and the toothbrushes had never been used. So, it is a problem getting the message across and actually putting it into action.

In 1963, the Royal Society of Health introduced the first Diploma in Dental Health Education, which I had invented, in this country. And they were so delighted and it was meant really more for school teachers, rather than dentists and possibly dental nurses. They wrote to the General Dental Council to say, you'll be pleased to know that we've just introduced this new Diploma in Dental Health Education, and sent the regulations. The General Dental Council wrote back to say we're very concerned about this development. Don't you know that dental health education is what dentists do? They wrote back to say that education is what teachers do.

It was six months later when the GDC made a pronouncement in the presidential address to say we've given this subject deep thought and we think dentists in practice know best and they should know when their dental nurse is sufficiently well taught to do dental health education on behalf of the dentist. And who knows, maybe there might be a Diploma in Dental Health Education to aid them in their endeavours. It's the whole profession that always lags, including the General Dental Council, behind a few leaders.

Dental therapists

Those of us who worked with auxiliaries, later therapists, realise the quality of the care which they provided. Of course, that wasn't surprising because they entered dentistry because they wanted to treat children. Most dentists just wanted to treat adults and children were a sort of by-word. And the other thing was that their course, the one-year clinical programme of a two-year course, was treatments with masses of fillings, and so the standard of the fillings that they were doing at the end of the course was far greater than most dental undergraduates were doing.

Those of us who worked with auxiliaries were amazed by the contribution they made and, at one time, I managed ten of them at the same time. And the production, the quantity and the quality were superb and when we had the Nuffield enquiry, looking at auxiliaries amongst several other things, they commented on the high standard of care which had been reported. And yet in their conclusions, they recommended closing the New Cross School, and of course this was all politics because the British Dental Association had got to them and said if they can't work in practice, they're not going to work anywhere.

The London Hospital, particularly Harry Aldred at the time, was quite clever. It said we agree that it's time for New Cross to be closed, but if you can see your way to keeping some form of auxiliary, we would like to train them. And of course, after New Cross was closed, the London went to the Ministry of Health and said, and it's published in the document, that it was prepared to train them, but alongside dentists. I don't know why they said that because some of the best hygienists in the country were trained in the services, not alongside dentists.

And the London Hospital, to its credit, picked it up and started a school, not of 60 a year, but of eight a year, and they trained them both as auxiliaries and hygienists so that they could work in practice, waiting for the day when they could work as therapists in practice, which of course now they can do. So that was very important because I think if the London hadn't held out at that time, there probably would be no auxiliaries, no therapists today.

There were a lot of issues in 1973, moving towards the reorganisation. There was the issue of dentistry related to medicine. If you study the history of dentistry, you'll see that there were always, the surgeons in particular, but doctors in general, saying we'd love to help you but we can't. What we found is, as we were fighting for a place for dentistry in the 1974 reorganisation, that in general doctors, including general medical practitioners, were supportive of dentistry, unless there was a shortage of money. And then when the chips were down, dentistry didn't get a look in. Part of the reason is that everything else in the NHS arises out of doctors, whether you're talking about speech therapies, psychotherapies, nursing or whatever. It all relies on the medical team and the dental team isn't part of it. So if you're short of money, the easiest thing you can do is to get rid of the dental bit and it doesn't make any difference to your own service.

My experience, and I'm sure other people's experience, is, a lot of general practitioners used to say to me, 'You know, I don't know what our patients would do if we didn't have a decent School Dental Service.' So they realised the benefits, particularly as the community service started making inroads, and it may have been different for me because inner London was different from other parts of the country, but there was bad dentistry going on in a lot of places in London, and they were grateful for the community service to take a lead and try to raise standards.

I think it's even more important now that salaried dentists get at these local medical practitioners who've got the money, because that's the trick everywhere, always has been. Who's got the money, and get in quick. No point in sitting back and moaning. And if they're the ones with the money, you've got to say to them, look, these are the advantages of having dentistry, whether it's care for the handicapped or whatever.

At the start of the National Health Service, there were many people who didn't think dentistry should be part of it. The British Dental Association was ambivalent. A lot of dentists, as well as doctors, couldn't earn a living in many parts of the country before the Health Service came in; there was not enough money to go round. We've already heard how, even after the Health Service, some people were coming in and saying, 'Take my teeth out.' But usually it didn't lead to any other treatment. The usual treatment was, hang on until pain is so bad, go to a dentist and have that tooth out. That was the common picture before the NHS.

There were reports showing that there was terrible dentistry around but what was shown clearly was, even if there were a better dental service, in many parts of the country, until there was education, it wouldn't matter because people still wouldn't seek dental treatment. And that was the biggest thing that had to be recognised from the beginning. There had to be education to show people it was worth preserving their teeth, alongside putting money into good dental care and good dental education.

That's when after the NHS started, round about the same time, when the dental schools expanded because it was a three-way process, the whole thing had to move ahead together. But we've seen all these and the biggest lesson is, with every reorganisation, there will be some disadvantages. Look for the advantages and look for the opportunities and those people who looked ahead and saw the opportunities, which were coming, were well placed to take those opportunities.

29. Nigel Williams.

Nigel qualified in 1973 and spent 13 years in general dental practice before joining the Community Dental Service. He talked to Stephen Simmons in 2012.

******

Joining the Community Dental Service

I joined the Community Dental Service in 1986, having been sacked from the general practice where I was an associate because I didn't cut 20 crowns a week. It was a lovely family practice, but then it was taken over by a real go-getter. I joined the CDS at that stage.

The district dental officer when I joined was Mr William Humpherson,[154] who was an extraordinary gentleman, very brilliant in his own way. And very far-sighted because I joined before HC(89)2,[155] but he was already saying to us all that we should treat more people with physical and mental difficulties and children, particularly with handicaps of different kinds.

Transfer away from a children's service

It was far-sighted but difficult for him because a lot of the dentists in the Community Dental Service at that time had only treated children and treated them very well, and for quite a long a period. So suddenly they were faced with converting to a totally different clientele, of whom they had very little experience. And this gradually came in with Mr Humpherson's encouragement. So when the change of the role came, there were quite a lot of seeds already sown in the mind, so it wasn't such a shock.

---

[154] See also: chapter 28, 30.

[155] HC(89)2 'The Future of the Community Dental Service' was a government circular in 1989 which said that the routine dental treatment of children should be redirected away from the community service to the general dental services. A government white paper 'Promoting Better Health' (Cm249,1987) had previously said that the community services would in future provide treatment for children and adults who experienced difficulty in getting treatment from General Dental Practitioners.

Hypnosis

Les Cheeseman taught me how to do relative analgesia.[156] He's an excellent teacher. But also, I went on a weekend course in Medical and Dental Hypnosis at the Royal Society of Medicine because it is now a fully recognised procedure. This was an extraordinary weekend where they carried out hypnotism on ourselves. Those who went, some of us were open-minded, some were absolutely certain it worked and a couple were certain it didn't and they wanted to prove it didn't.

We were given an introductory group relaxation therapy and all during the day this chap had said, 'No, doesn't work, doesn't work.' During the afternoon session the lecturer said to us, 'Would you like to look at him?' He was completely out. During the morning, they'd implanted in his mind a signal and the lecturer gave that in the afternoon and he went totally relaxed, just like that, and to sleep. When we brought him back to reality, he was totally convinced.

Dental Therapists

During my years in the Community Dental Service, we had two dental therapists who worked for us. One was absolutely superb, a lady called Ruth Lovering. I'm ashamed to say I think her dentistry was probably a bit better than mine, and her way, with particularly challenged children, was absolutely superb. The other therapist we had, unfortunately, wasn't so good, because about two years after she joined us, we found out that she couldn't actually recognise caries. That became very difficult because, how do you handle that situation? But in the end, I think we persuaded her that, through her qualification, she could be a hygienist as well and that should be the line she went down.

Orthodontics

In Croydon, we were very lucky in that we had two large orthodontic practices, one of which was run by a chap called Pat McDonough and now is run by his son Tim. The quality of service they gave was fantastic and needless to say, being Community Dental Service, we had to refer quite a lot of very difficult behaviour children to them and they were wonderful, and also a lot of 'normal' children who were unhappy with slight defects of their appearance. I believe with the new regulations within the contract the orthodontist is not allowed to treat children with relatively minor discrepancies. The sad thing was that the orthodontist had no choice but to only do those children privately. So suddenly you

---

[156] See also chapter 11, 28, 30.

had a situation where the rich could afford their children to look lovely and poorer people couldn't.

Education

When I joined the CDS, my two senior dental officers had both been general dental practitioners themselves before they joined, so they had that background, and both of them were common-sense people. They had a wealth of experience within themselves, which they kindly shared with me and guided me a lot when I first joined. Later on William Humpherson[157] encouraged me to join an MSc course at King's run by Professor Stanley Gelbier. Now I only completed part of that course but I saw all sorts of aspects of dental life and sociological life during that, which has always stood me in good stead.

Then I transferred over to do the Diploma in Dental Public Health, with John Bulman.[158] And suddenly I was in educational heaven because being the type of person I am I learn by rote and that was exactly how John Bulman did it. I thought that was wonderful. Some years later I came to a CCCDS[159] lecture where a gentleman, who I will call a dry fingered dentist from the Midlands, was lecturing. He had set up a new career pathway which he thought all CDS people should go through, a lot of which was academic, for which I have great respect, but not much was clinical. Three quarters of the way through his lecture he said, 'And of course, now we don't want any general dental service rubbish in the CDS.' I've never been so upset in all my life and I stood up at the back and called the chairman to attention, I said, 'Will you ask the speaker to withdraw that comment?' And he wouldn't. Four of us walked out. We went down to the pub. I was genuinely in tears and they were almost in tears because I think a breadth of experience before you join the CDS is very valuable.

Audit became a very fashionable thing all of a sudden, and many management consultants were hired by the Department of Health to lecture us on how to do it. But in fact, it's a very simple thing. You look at what you're doing and you study it and attempt to improve. I think in Croydon we did a pretty good job of that. It wasn't very esoteric; it wasn't highly statistical, but it was practical.

---

[157] District Dental Officer.
[158] Reader and Honorary Consultant in Dental Public Health Eastman Dental Institute.
[159] Central Committee for Community Dental Services.

Reorganisations

I went through a whole series of reorganisations when Community Trusts were first formed. When it was first formed, the Croydon Community Trust was quite small, led by a wonderful woman call Judy Hargadon as the chief executive, who pulled the Trust together. She knew everybody's name and every lunchtime she would visit a different clinic. You always had access to her.

But as time went by and different reorganisations came in, the administrative department became bigger and bigger. It ended up with two administrators, highly paid, appointed to study our audits. And then they called a group of the head of audit for each department to criticise each other's audits before the audit would finally be accepted by the Authority. I thought that was ridiculous. Profession is a dirty word, but if we were doing audits, we were quite capable. The chief executive could just glance at it and it would be fine.

I trained to do the BASCD surveys in Birmingham.[160] At lunchtime somebody was talking about fluoride in Birmingham. They actually had to bus the kids in from outside Birmingham, so that there was some caries for us to look at because the children in Birmingham, from every social stratum, didn't have any caries.[161]

When I first started work in the Health Service, if I went to somebody's retirement, they were usually in tears because they loved it so much and the last thing they wanted to do was to retire. In the last ten years, every retirement party I've gone to, the person retiring has been skipping with joy. Also, when I see them a few years later, they look ten years younger than when they retired. I know that working in community dentistry with challenged people is very stressful. There are enormous rewards, but most nights I'd have a job getting to sleep, worrying about the patient I was going to see the next day, and I think that's part of it. Also, the changes in the Health Service, and the administration and the accountability, I think that increased the stress. But I certainly I enjoyed my career.

---

[160] British Association for the Study of Community Dentistry.
[161] See Chapter 23.

30. Leslie Cheeseman

Leslie worked as a surgery assistant during National Service which inspired him to be a dentist. His long career started with many years in general practice before he joined the schools and subsequently community services. He spoke with Stephen Simmons in 2012.[162]

******

Childhood memory of the dentist 1932

On my entry to infants' school in 1931 at age four, I was referred to the School Dental Service, as it then was, and I vividly remember having attended a GA session, where I had all eight deciduous molar teeth extracted. My memory was that I was given a gas anaesthetic, but I don't believe I was ever sufficiently unconscious. It was a horrific experience, as was the severe post extraction haemorrhage afterwards. From that point on, I had a fear of dentistry.

Perhaps two years passed and the school dentist came, and I was recommended to have some fillings placed in permanent teeth and my mother signed the form and I duly went to the clinic, where the same dentist as before was on duty. He was, no doubt, a very efficient dentist, technically, but he didn't know how to cope with patients and pain control didn't come into the situation at all. Now we probably all remember having a permanent molar drilled and filled, without locals, a horrific experience. The man couldn't possibly finish my six-year-old molar because I had memories of the gas session before and I remember this man was just inflicting pain and so the uncompleted cavity was left open to the elements. From that point on, I never wanted any dental care again. So, it's quite remarkable that I eventually became a dentist.

Inspired to dentistry as a surgery assistant in the RAF

Now, the reason I became a dentist was that I was shanghaied into the Air Force Dental Branch at age 17. I was under air crew training and

---

[162] See: Leslie Cheeseman BEM: dentist and cricket umpire. Gelbier S, Dental Historian 2012; 56: 90-94

they didn't want air crews anymore, so I was re-mustered compulsorily, to the RAF Dental Branch. We had a dental inspection and the state of my permanent dentition was a lot worse than it was six years earlier so I needed extensive restoration treatment.

But I could see that the chap that I was working for, as a Dental Surgery Assistant, a Flight Lieutenant Hardy, was quite a different person to the school dentist because he used locals, and he administered pain control. And that really changed my attitude completely. From that point on I was interested in following dentistry because he removed pain to prevent fear, and it did precisely that, and that changed my whole life.

At that time the Air Force Dental Branch actually invented dental hygienists.[163] I don't know if that's generally known. Sir William Kelsey Fry introduced the grade as a pilot scheme, which was quite successful.

Relative analgesia

One of the most significant differences that I found between the two services, because I was in general practice before I became a community dental officer, was that when I joined the Community Dental Service, preventive dentistry had a much greater emphasis than it ever did in general dental practice.

Relative analgesia made a significant difference in how dental phobics and the mentally and physically handicapped people who were untreatable before in the conscious state, could be treated.

It wasn't until I joined the Community Dental Service full-time in 1977 that Mr Humpherson[164] suggested I attend a course on relative analgesia provided by one of his colleagues from the South West Thames Regional Dental Officers Group, Mr Bristow. The tutor was a man from Harrogate, a senior dental officer whose name I've forgotten. But I went on this course and was astounded at what a difference it made. It was a clinical course, and I developed a major interest. But I don't think it was known generally in this country before 1978. It made a tremendous difference to the quality of care provided by me, personally. It provided a fail-safe and highly efficient form of conscious sedation, allowing both protective swallow and cough reflexes to remain intact, enabling me to provide hassle-free care to those patients who were former dental phobics, plus those who presented with physical or learning disabilities.

---

[163] The RAF didn't invent hygienists, they were in the USA decades before See Chapter 10.
[164] District Dental Officer, see chapter 28, 29.

Its major benefits were to reduce exposure to the risks associated with general anaesthesia, to be suitable for administration to patients of all ages without the pre-operative necessity of ensuring the patient had an empty stomach and, finally, enabling them to be cared for as ambulant out-patients. Once patients became 'converted' to the technique, there was seldom any difficulty in arranging for them to accept repeated appointments and they never cancelled or failed to attend those subsequently arranged without good reason.

I know that in the States and in the European low countries they used relative analgesia as opposed to GA. In fact, I remember the Festival of Britain, in 1951. I was a fourth-year student at Guy's, and the Dental Society had a group of Danish dental undergraduates over as guests. They wanted to see a GA outpatients' exodontia session, because in Denmark the administration of GA, in relation to dentistry, was prohibited at all levels. But instead of having GA, they had relative analgesia, which we didn't understand at that time, as the knowledge and practice of the RA technique was unknown to us. We tended to pooh pooh it. It had not been introduced to us by our tutors and therefore the technique had little or no credibility for us.

Dental Auxiliaries

The standard of care provided by auxiliaries I found in my personal experience to be absolutely exemplary. They were dedicated individuals, but more than that, I think their standard of care rivalled that provided by dental officers. This may have been because of the professional supervision that had to be applied to each patient, that the dentist used to have to prescribe the treatment and, of course, he would see the child again. So you would actually see the quality of care which was being provided. And that may have been a primary reason it was so good.

But there was no similar experience in general dental practice; nobody else witnessed the sort of work I was turning out unless I happened to be reviewed by a regional dental officer, and I never had a problem with them. But the point was there was an informal policing of dental auxiliaries' work by the prescribing dentist, which was only to the good. The first dental auxiliary qualified in 1962, New Cross opened in 1960 and it closed in 1983.[165] So it was open for 23 years.

---

[165] The New Cross School for Dental Auxiliaries.

Orthodontics in School Dental Service

There's been a significant change over the years in the diagnosis of malocclusion and the treatment of it. One thing which was positive about school inspections was that one could pick up early malocclusions in certain people, like just a simple incisor inside the bite, which one could rectify fairly quickly, without too much orthodontic knowledge or technique.

It is worth noting the parents, who following the CDS recommendation for the need for orthodontic treatment, found that many of their own General Dental Practitioners were not interested in uptake of the orthodontic intervention recommended. The reason for this was unclear. It may have been because the problem of correction was outside their orthodontic skills, but it was puzzling why they did not make referrals to specialist orthodontic colleagues known to work in general NHS practice.

Many of the latter would only accept those in need of orthodontic care on a private basis. Thus, a two-tier system developed whereby children with affluent parents received treatment and those from poorer backgrounds did not. I understand that annual inspections of children at school are now no longer mandatory and I think this is a pity since evidence of incipient malocclusions (and indeed, other incipient forms of dental pathology) in non-regular attenders may no longer be identified at the most appropriate times for correction.

There came a stage when funding became tight, that was when the responsibility for the wellbeing of the Community Dental Service was transferred from the Local Authorities to the Health Authorities. I confirm that with my experience, the only safeguard happened when the Health and Safety at Work Act came in.[166] That made a tremendous difference. I could get quite a lot of clout, because of that Act, in getting money I couldn't get hold of before.

The formation of the Health Service itself was a major change and the nature of dental services needed significant change. For instance, I've already recounted my own miserable appreciation of dentistry early on as a child, but I never remember seeing my mother and father other than with full upper and lower, vulcanite dentures. And I think that was more or less true of most of the adult population in the 1930s, the 1940s and

---

[166] Health and Safety at Work etc. Act 1974.

maybe the early 1950s. I think everyone in my age group remembers virtually every adult person wearing vulcanite dentures with porcelain teeth of the same shade. There've been tremendous changes in prosthesis over my working lifetime.

Prevention in general practice and community service

I would like to build further on the differences between the services provided by General Dental Practitioners and the Community Dental Officers. Prior to the late 1970s, I spent over 20 years as a General Dental Practitioner before the first of several NHS re-organisations were made, when I then switched to become a Senior Dental Officer in the Community Dental Service.

One of the major differences between the two was that the practice of preventive dentistry within the Community Dental Service had a much greater emphasis than it ever did in general dental practice. We attended copious meetings where both disciplines were represented and it became clear that General Dental Practitioners were at least suspicious, or more often antagonistic, towards the beneficial concept of preventive dentistry.

It has to be appreciated that at the time, General Dental Practitioners were handsomely remunerated by performing items of service that were treatment orientated and it was perceived not to be in their financial interest to have anything introduced that might negate their need to 'drill and fill'. Hence their disinterest in most aspects of preventive dentistry, which did not feature in the Dental Estimates Board Scale of Fees. Most of us who have served within the Community Dental Service know well the long-term beneficial effects of a major reduction in caries experience which follows the introduction of fluoride to water supplies, the application of topical fluoride gels or varnishes, the commercial introduction of the fluoride ion to toothpastes and the selected low dose medication prescribed to young infants. All of these were generally anathema to the, primarily caries interested, General Dental Practitioner.

The beneficial effect of introducing fluoride has been confirmed by the massive reduction of population DMF [167] scores over the past 40 years, highlighted by the comparative results of successive dental surveys that were undertaken by the Community Dental Service during this period.

---

[167] Decayed, missing or filled teeth.

Introducing adhesive fissure sealants around this time also made significant reductions to the incidence of occlusal carious attack and some General Dental Practitioners were not slow to appreciate that there was potential financial benefit in promoting these as additional sources to their private income, because they were not included in the range of treatments approved for payment by the Dental Estimates Board.

A 'knock-on' effect of the reduction of caries experience became highlighted in the results of successive adult dental surveys made throughout this period. They have shown that a reduction in the young has resulted in an increasing number of adults remaining dentate throughout their lifetimes, with a reduced requirement for the prosthetic provision of full upper and lower dentures. In population terms, there has been a sea-change in the overall improvement of dental health. My interest in preventive dentistry came alive when I joined the Community Dental Service and the reduction in caries experience because of the introduction of fluoride in its various forms has been the single most cause of improvement in dental health of the community at large and has been, truly amazing.

John McLean

John McLean was a prominent dentist and material scientist who made significant advances in his research into dental materials, which he combined with private dental practice.

John was born in Cardiff in 1925 and was educated at Westminster Abbey Choir School. He studied dentistry at Guy's hospital, where he won several prizes, and qualified with the LDS Royal College of Surgeons diploma.

His interest in material science started as an undergraduate and after qualification he combined private dental practice in central London with materials research. He taught at Guy's hospital dental school for a short time and later was a lecturer in dental materials at the Eastman Dental Institute.

He became a clinical consultant to the Laboratory of the Government Chemist. He researched self-curing acrylic resins, silicone impression materials, and high strength ceramics, vacuum fired ceramics, and bonded porcelain and glass ionomer cements.

He wrote many papers on materials and the standard textbook on dental ceramics.[168] He was president of the British Society of Restorative Dentistry, the British Dental Association and became an elected member of the General Dental Council.

John McLean died in 2009 and among several bequests he made was one to the British Dental Association which was used to finance the John McLean archive: a living history of dentistry, which comprises witness seminars and oral history interviews.[169]

---

[168] The Science and Art of Dental Ceramics.
[169] Creating the John McLean Archive: a living history of Dentistry. Nairn Wilson, Rachel Bairsto, Stanley Gelbier. Dental Historian 2012 July (56) 70-72.
See: John McLean . OBE His Life and Times. Peter Frost. Dental Historian 2007. Jan (44) 5-19.

The Interviewers

Austin Banner, Malcolm Bishop, Janet Heath, Frank Holloway,
Ros Levenson, Mark McCutcheon, Judith Painter, Sophie Riches,
Pam Royle, Andrew Sadler, Stephen Simmons, Brian Williams
Margaret Wilson.

Acknowledgements

I am indebted to the subjects for their time in agreeing to be interviewed.
Rachel Bairsto, the head of museum services and archives at the British
Dental Association who administers the John McLean history archive
and arranges the professional transcription of the audio recordings.

Sophie Riches initially set up and administered the archive. The British
Orthodontic Society owns the copyright of the interview of Ron
Broadway that was conducted by Sophie and Austin Banner and allowed
me to use the transcription. The British Dental Association own the
copyright of the other original recordings and transcriptions and allowed
the use the material and image on the front cover.

The libraries of the British Dental Association and Royal Society of
Medicine hold a wealth of historical books and journals which I have
referred to.

My wife Maralyn has line edited the text and given me good council in
content editing.

Also by Andrew Sadler

Dentist on the Ward: An Introduction to Oral and Maxillofacial Surgery
and Medicine for Core Trainees in Dentistry – *Andrew Sadler and Leo
Cheng*

Core Oral Surgery for Dental Students: Essential Knowledge for
Qualifying Dental Examinations – *Andrew Sadler and Edmund Bailey*

The Making of British Oral and Maxillofacial Surgery:
Voices of Pioneers and Witnesses to its Evolution from Hospital
Dentistry – *Andrew Sadler*

Index

www.ingramcontent.com/pod-product-compliance
Lightning Source LLC
Chambersburg PA
CBHW071332210326
41597CB00015B/1431